Diseases of the Ear, Nose & Throat in Children

Diseases of the Ear, Nose & Throat in Children

AN INTRODUCTION AND PRACTICAL GUIDE

Raymond W Clarke BA, BSc., DCH, FRCS, FRCS(ORL)

Paediatric Otolaryngologist
Alder Hey and University of Liverpool
Liverpool, UK

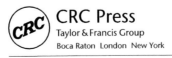

CRC Press
Taylor & Francis Group
Boca Raton London New York

CRC Press is an imprint of the
Taylor & Francis Group, an **informa** business

First edition published 2023
by CRC Press
6000 Broken Sound Parkway NW, Suite 300, Boca Raton, FL 33487-2742

and by CRC Press
4 Park Square, Milton Park, Abingdon, Oxon, OX14 4RN

CRC Press is an imprint of Taylor & Francis Group, LLC

Library of Congress Cataloging-in-Publication Data

Names: Clarke, Ray (Raymond) author.
Title: Diseases of the ear, nose & throat in children : an introduction and practical guide / Raymond W. Clarke.
 Other titles: Diseases of the ear, nose and throat in children
Description: First edition. | Boca Raton : CRC Press, 2022. | Includes bibliographical references and index. |
 Summary: "An essential introduction to the clinical examination, treatment and surgical procedures for children
 with diseases of the ear, nose and throat. This book encompasses the conditions most commonly encountered in the
 emergency setting, on the ward and in the outpatient clinic. With its highly practical approach and step-by-step guidance,
 this book will be invaluable for all surgical trainees studying for higher postgraduate examinations in ENT, as well as an
 essential guide for otorhinolaryngologists, primary care practitioners and specialist ENT nurses in the early years of
 training"— Provided by publisher.
Identifiers: LCCN 2021062701 (print) | LCCN 2021062702 (ebook) | ISBN 9781138579422 (hardback) |
 ISBN 9781138579347 (paperback) | ISBN 9780429019128 (ebook)
Subjects: MESH: Otorhinolaryngologic Diseases | Child | Emergencies | Otorhinolaryngologic Surgical Procedures
Classification: LCC RF32 (print) | LCC RF32 (ebook) | NLM WV 140 | DDC 617.5/1083—dc23/eng/20220328
LC record available at https://lccn.loc.gov/2021062701
LC ebook record available at https://lccn.loc.gov/2021062702

ISBN: 978-1-138-57942-2 (hbk)
ISBN: 978-1-138-57934-7 (pbk)
ISBN: 978-0-429-01912-8 (ebk)

DOI: 10.1201/9780429019128

Typeset in Minion Pro
by Apex CoVantage, LLC

CONTENTS

PREFACE

Paediatric otolaryngology is a growing discipline with a large and increasingly complex body of knowledge to guide specialist practitioners. The subspecialty is already well covered by some excellent textbooks and reference works. The general ORL doctor, with a mixed adult and child practice, is less well served and often bemoans the lack of a short, easy-to-read account of the main disorders in children. I hope this little book fills that gap.

I have focused in the main on common conditions unique to children or where the presentation and management are different in children than in their adult counterparts. This has meant leaving much material out, for example in otology – including implantation otology, now a very large part of paediatric practice – where there is already very good material available in the standard adult texts.

I hope candidates for the main postgraduate examinations (e.g. the UEMS Boards, and the UK Intercollegiate fellowship) will have enough revision material to satisfy the curriculum, that the established generalist in ORL will find enough in the way of advice regarding investigation and management of the common conditions to support them in their day-to-day work looking after children, and that the newcomer to ORL will be motivated to learn more about paediatric aspects of our specialty.

I have deliberately kept the chapters short, with summaries of the main points, and a very small number of references as readers now have near-universal recourse to multiple up-to-date online sources of knowledge. Throughout, I have tried to give sound advice that will be of use in the clinical situation, much of it based on long personal experience.

Working with children, families, colleagues and trainees in paediatric ORL has been a lifelong pleasure and I hope this short text will stimulate others to share that joy.

R.W. Clarke
Paediatric ORL Dept.
Royal Liverpool Children's Hospital
Alder Hey
Liverpool, UK

Honorary Professor
University of Liverpool

ACKNOWLEDGEMENTS

Thanks to Miranda Bromage and her team at Taylor & Francis for seeing this book to completion. Becky Freeman, Daina Habdankaite and Nora Naughton provided immense support and patience as the manuscript developed. Sue Tyler drew several new illustrations, and Dr Shiv Avula helped with the radiological images. Dr Sudhira Ratnayake advised on the audiology content, and Ms Ann-Louise McDermott helped with the chapter on COVID-19.

Many of the figures are borrowed from Scott Brown's *Otolaryngology Head and Neck Surgery*, 8th Edition, Taylor & Francis 2018, and I am grateful to the chapter authors for providing high-quality images.

ABBREVIATIONS

ABC — aspiration biopsy cytology
ABI — auditory brainstem implant
ABR — auditory brainstem response
ABRS — acute bacterial rhinosinusitis
AC — air conduction
AD — auditory dysynchrony
ADD — attention deficit disorder
ADHD — attention deficit hyperactivity disorder
AGP — aerosol-generating procedure
AHI — apnoea/hypopnoea index
AIDS — acquired immunodeficiency syndrome
ALTB — acute laryngotracheobronchitis
AMT — appropriate medical treatment
ANSD — auditory neuropathy spectrum disorder
AOM — acute otitis media
APAGBI — Association of Paediatric Anaesthetists of Great Britain and Ireland
APLS — Advanced Paediatric Life Support™
AR — allergic rhinitis / allergic rhinoconjunctivitis / allergic rhinosinusitis
ARS — acute rhinosinusitis
ASD — autistic spectrum disorder
ATM — atypical mycobacteria
BAHA — bone-anchored hearing aid
BAPO — British Association for Paediatric Otolaryngology
BC — bone conduction
BCHD — bone-conducting hearing device
BOA — behavioural observation audiometry
BPAP — bilevel positive airway pressure
BPCHI — bilateral permanent childhood hearing impairment
BPPV — benign paroxysmal positional vertigo
BPVC — benign paroxysmal vertigo of childhood

CF — cystic fibrosis
CHAOS — congenital high airway obstruction syndrome
CI — cochlear implant
CMV — cytomegalovirus
COM — chronic otitis media
CPAP — continuous positive airway pressure
CRP — C-reactive protein
CRS — chronic rhinosinusitis
CSOM — chronic suppurative otitis media
CT — computed tomography
CTR — cricotracheal resection
CWD — canal wall down
CWU — canal wall up
CYP — children and young people
DISE — drug-induced sleep endoscopy
DNS — deep neck space
DSA — Down's Syndrome Association
EBV — Epstein Barr virus
ED — emergency department
ENT — ear, nose and throat
EPOS2020 — European Position Paper on Rhinosinusitis and Nasal Polyps 2020
ET — endotracheal
EXIT — *ex utero* intrapartum treatment
FESS — functional endoscopic sinus surgery
FFP — filtering face-piece
FII — Fabricated or Induced Illness
FNA — fine-needle aspiration
GABHS — group A beta-haemolytic *Streptococcus pyogenes*
GI — gastrointestinal
GMC — General Medical Council
HCW — healthcare workers
HDU — high-dependency unit
Hib — *Haemophilus influenza* B
HIV — human immunodeficiency virus
HL — hearing loss
HPV — human papillomavirus
IgE — immunoglobulin E

INCS	intranasal corticosteroid	PPE	personal protective equipment
IV	intravenous	PSA	pleomorphic salivary adenoma
JOF	juvenile ossifying fibroma	PSG	polysomnography
JORRP	juvenile-onset recurrent respiratory papillomatosis	PTA	pure-tone audiometry
		RAOM	recurrent acute otitis media
LCH	Langerhans cell histiocytosis	RARS	recurrent acute rhinosinusitis
LMA	laryngeal mask airway	RCoA	Royal College of Anaesthetists
LTR	laryngotracheal reconstruction	RCPCH	Royal College of Paediatrics and Child Health
MDT	multidisciplinary team		
MEI	middle ear implant	REM	rapid eye movement
MMR	mumps, measles, rubella	RRP	recurrent respiratory papillomatosis
MRI	magnetic resonance imaging		
NAI	non-accidental injury	RSV	respiratory syncytial virus
NF2	neurofibromatosis type 2	SALT	speech and language therapist
NO	nitrous oxide	SARS-CoV-2	severe acute respiratory syndrome coronavirus 2
NORD	National Organization for Rare Disorders		
		SCBU	special care baby unit
NPA	nasopharyngeal airway	SCIT	subcutaneous immunotherapy
NSAID	non-steroidal anti-inflammatory drug	SDB	sleep-disordered breathing
NTM	non-tuberculous mycobacteria	SGS	subglottic stenosis
OAE	otoacoustic emission	SIGN	Scottish Intercollegiate Guidelines Network
OME	otitis media with effusion		
OR	operating room	SLIT	sublingual immunotherapy
ORL	otorhinolaryngology	SSD	single-sided deafness
OSA	obstructive sleep apnoea	THRIVE	trans-nasal humidified rapid insufflation ventilatory exchange
PCD	primary ciliary dyskinesia		
PCHI	permanent childhood hearing impairment hearing	TOF	tracheo-oesophageal fistula
		TSH	thyroid stimulating hormone
PCHI	permanent congenital hearing impairment	UK	United Kingdom
		VACTERL	vertebral, anal, cardiac, tracheal, renal and limb
PCHR	Personal Child Health Record		
PCR	polymerase chain reaction	VRA	visual reinforcement audiometry
PEWS	paediatric early warning signs	WHO/REAL	World Health Organization/ Revised European American Lymphoma
PICU	paediatric intensive care unit		
PONV	postoperative nausea and vomiting		

1

INTRODUCTION

Specialists in otorhinolaryngology (ORL) have looked after children since the beginnings of the specialty. Children's hospitals and dedicated paediatricians came to the fore from the early twentieth century onwards. It was clear that ORL surgeons were essential to the care of children and the subspecialty of paediatric otolaryngology gradually came into being. Paediatric ORL specialists work mainly in children's hospitals – or in the children's sections of general hospitals – and focus on problems such as airway pathology, congenital head and neck disorders, benign and malignant neck disease and ORL issues in children with complex medical conditions. Most general ORL specialists will also see large numbers of children with tonsil and adenoid disease, obstructive sleep apnoea, otitis media and congenital and acquired hearing loss. Whatever healthcare setting you work in, it is important to have a good grounding in the basics of ear, nose and throat (ENT) pathologies in children and in the general principles that make for optimum care of sick children and their families.

ORL SERVICES FOR CHILDREN

Paediatric otolaryngologists look after 'special problems or special children, or both, in a special institution' (Bluestone, 1995).

Services for children and young people (CYP) can be delivered in multiple ways in different health systems. In the UK and much of Europe and beyond, most ORL specialists have a mixed adult and paediatric practice. A small, but increasing, number devote most or all of their professional time to looking after children. Tertiary and advanced care is provided in designated children's hospitals (**Figure 1.1**) with ready access to other specialists, to paediatric intensive care units (PICUs) and to anaesthesiologists who work exclusively with children and have a great deal of expertise in the perioperative care of sick children. Some of the larger general hospitals have paediatric sections which include these facilities, and most hospitals where ORL specialists work will look after children with the more common ORL pathologies, but typically not the very young or very sick children who may need PICU.

ORL doctors perform more surgical interventions in children than any other surgical discipline. We can be powerful advocates for improved care of children and should be to the fore when services are planned or reconfigured.

Children are best seen in dedicated clinics where there are no adult patients, and with good audiology testing facilities. This is easily accomplished in

DOI: 10.1201/9780429019128-1

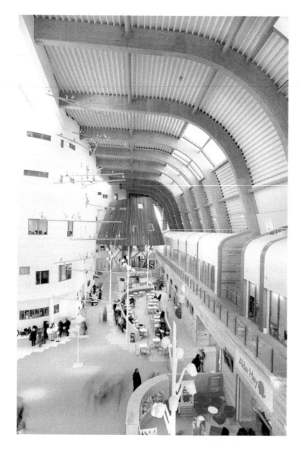

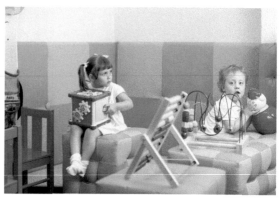

Figure 1.2 A 'child-friendly' clinic waiting room.

Figure 1.1 The foyer, Alder Hey Children's Hospital, Liverpool.

ideally with a trained and registered children's nurse in charge (**Figure 1.2**).

Children are best cared for as close to home as possible, in an environment suited to their needs. Despite the desirability of looking after children and families in a local setting, children with complex conditions, or who need highly specialised interventions, are better managed in a regional centre where resources and skills are concentrated. This will necessitate good communication and liaison strategies between different hospitals with carefully planned arrangements for transfer and for safe transport, particularly in emergency situations. Many hospitals now have a 'retrieval' service whereby a sick child can be resuscitated and stabilised, including endotracheal (ET) intubation where needed, by a skilled team before being transferred for definitive care to a specialist centre.

children's hospitals but needs more careful planning in a general hospital. Clinics and waiting areas need to be 'child-friendly' with suitable toys, paper and pens, and facilities for siblings and nursing mothers,

PERIOPERATIVE CARE

■ Surgical lists

Operating lists for children ideally should be for children only, i.e. dedicated children's lists. This has become the norm in many health systems, but it can be difficult to schedule in a mixed adult and children's hospital and is dependent on local funding arrangements and resources. Operating room

staff need to be suitably trained; the anaesthesiology and recovery teams in particular should have expertise and training in looking after children. Different national societies and organisations will have their own guidelines. Where it is deemed safe, and the surgical and anaesthetic teams have agreed arrangements, 'day-case' or 'same-day' surgery is generally preferred, but clearly this depends on issues such as transport, home facilities, and local customs and expectation. Children who need an overnight stay or admission to wards are best looked after in a children's rather than a mixed adult and child ward.

▮ Anaesthesia

Good rapport and mutual understanding between surgeon and anaesthetist are especially important in children's ORL procedures. Both surgeon and anaesthetist 'share' the airway, which is often narrow and already compromised, especially in a very young child. The two methods of providing an anaesthetic for a child are essentially *simple anaesthesia* and *balanced anaesthesia*.

'Simple' anaesthesia involves administering a single agent to induce unconsciousness and lack of movement in response to surgical stimulation. The agent is typically a vapour (e.g. halothane, or more often sevoflurane), but intravenous (IV) agents such as Propofol and the benzodiazepines (Midazolam) are increasingly popular. The widespread use of the laryngeal mask airway (LMA) permits easy administration of vapours, including air and oxygen, during anaesthesia without the use of an ET tube or a cumbersome hand-held face mask. This has made simple anaesthesia more widely available for many 'minor' ORL procedures such as myringotomy and grommet insertion. Some surgeons and anaesthetists now use the LMA for adenotonsillectomy (**Figure 1.3**).

The widespread use of oil-based local anaesthetic agents – 'magic cream' such as Ametop® (Smith & Nephew) or EMLA® (AstraZeneca) – applied to the skin over a suitable vein before venepuncture has made IV injections to induce anaesthesia far less frightening. A small number of children will need a 'pre-med', typically a benzodiazepine such as Midazolam, but this may prolong the recovery period ('hangover') and is best avoided if possible.

'Balanced' anaesthesia involves the use of separate drugs to induce loss of consciousness, paralysis, and cardiovascular control and analgesia. An anaesthetic agent, a muscle relaxant and an opiate are usually

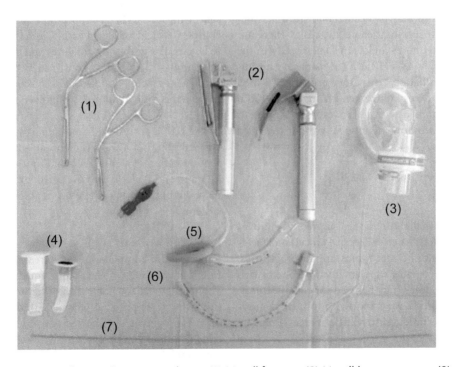

Figure 1.3 Equipment for paediatric anaesthesia: (1) Magill forceps, (2) Magill laryngoscopes, (3) ventilating facemask, (4) Guedel (oropharyngeal) airways, (5) LMA, (6) ET tube, (7) bougie.

combined. The paralysed patient will need to be ventilated, either by the anaesthetist by hand or via a mechanical ventilator. More sophisticated monitoring and awareness of the possibility of hypoxia are required, but balanced anaesthesia permits longer and more invasive procedures in younger and frailer patients, with reduced postoperative morbidity.

Anaesthesia and perioperative care of children undergoing laryngo-tracheoscopy, often with some form of open or endoscopic surgery to the larynx or trachea, require particularly close cooperation between surgeon and anaesthetist. Usually, the child will need to be breathing spontaneously, ideally without an ET tube obstructing the surgeon's access to the glottis and subglottis. The ET tube can rest in the pharynx and, if the surgeon requires access to the trachea and bronchi for a longer period, a ventilating bronchoscope permits safe and prolonged administration of oxygen and anaesthetic vapours. Topical anaesthesia (Xylocaine spray) to the mucosa of the glottis makes for reduced laryngospasm, but gentle and controlled introduction of telescopes and instruments also helps in this regard. Occasionally, a short period of apnoea may be needed and the anaesthetist will want to 'pre-oxygenate' the child. There has been increased interest of late in some centres in the technique known as THRIVE (trans-nasal humidified rapid insufflation ventilatory exchange), which involves the delivery of oxygen via high-flow nasal cannulas combined with IV anaesthesia to permit an extended 'window' of apnoea without the need for an ET tube.

▌ Analgesia

Adequate and well-chosen analgesia greatly improves the outcome in children's surgery. Paracetamol (acetaminophen) is sufficient for most minor procedures. Intraoperative opiates supplemented by one or two postoperative doses may be used for tonsillectomy, but local protocols vary and, with improved modern surgical techniques, very little analgesia may be required.

Postoperative nausea and vomiting (PONV) may be worsened by the use of opiates and can make for a very unhappy experience for both parent and child. Again, protocols vary but many units use prophylactic agents such as ondansetron (a serotonin antagonist) to reduce this troublesome complication. There is now good evidence that one single intraoperative dose of a corticosteroid (dexamethasone) improves PONV.

Codeine is no longer appropriate in young children due to the risk of catastrophic idiosyncratic reactions, especially in children with obstructive sleep apnoea (OSA) and should only be used with extreme caution in older children and adolescents. Non-steroidal anti-inflammatory drugs (NSAIDs, e.g. diclofenac, ibuprofen) are now widely used and are safe and effective despite some concerns that they may increase the incidence of postoperative bleeding.

▌ Consent in children

Every medical intervention requires the full agreement of the patient, but children may not have the capacity and understanding ('competence') to evaluate the benefits and risks of a procedure, and 'consent' will need to be given on their behalf. This is a complex ethical and legal area. Clinicians will need to be familiar with the guidelines and arrangements in their jurisdiction and as outlined by their national medical regulatory bodies. It is, of course, wise to involve the child at all times wherever possible.

In the UK, a person with 'parental responsibility' – typically but not always the parent – can give consent on behalf of a child. A 'child' in this context in England and Wales is a young person up to the age of 16 years, but this definition varies across healthcare systems.

A child under the age of 16 years may well be able to understand the implications of a treatment strategy. In UK law, a child who has 'sufficient understanding and intelligence to enable him or her to understand fully what is proposed' is termed 'Gillick competent' or 'Fraser competent'. The decision as to whether the child is 'Gillick competent' rests with the clinician, so you could decide that a teenager, for example, undergoing a tonsillectomy can give their own 'consent'. It is best practice to involve the parents at all times.

The 'Montgomery' legal judgment in the UK has clarified the requirements for consent even further. Essentially, the judgment of the courts places a duty on the clinician to explore in detail the patient's (or in the case of a child, the responsible adult's) likely assessment of the impact of the benefits and risks of an intervention *in his or her particular circumstances.*

In other words, the discussion regarding treatment options needs to be open, frank and customised to *that* individual patient's needs and priorities. An example might be the possible impact of a change in voice, which could be of great importance to a child who was a keen singer but of less importance to another child.

ORGANISATIONS AND SOCIETIES

As paediatric ORL progressed, it became clear that ORL and allied specialists needed to meet, exchange ideas, foster education and advocate for children, their families and the professionals who look after them. There are now several national and international societies focusing on paediatric ORL, with excellent educational and information resources. The Royal College of Paediatrics and Child Health (RCPCH) in the United Kingdom (UK) provides a wealth of resources – many available to non-members – and most of the various national ORL societies now have a section focusing on ORL issues in children (**Box 1.1**)

Box 1.1 Organisations and societies

American Society of Pediatric
   Otolaryngology: https://aspo.us
British Association for Paediatric
   Otolaryngology: https://www.bapo.
   co.uk
Confederation of European
   Otorhinolaryngology – Head and Neck
   Surgery: https://www.ceorlhns.org
European Society of Pediatric
   Otorhinolaryngology: http://espo.eu.com
Royal College of Paediatrics and Child
   Health: https://www.rcpch.ac.uk

KEY POINTS

- Children are best treated in dedicated clinics, with appropriately trained staff.
- Audiology staff, soundproof testing rooms and facilities for tympanometry are an integral part of the ORL clinic.
- Children's surgery should be performed during 'children's' theatre lists, with an experienced children's anaesthetist and support staff.
- Codeine is no longer appropriate as an analgesic agent in young children.
- 'Parental responsibility' varies in different jurisdictions but, in the UK, it essentially includes the child's mother, and the child's father if he is married to the child's mother or named on the birth certificate.
- Check local arrangements for 'looked after' or 'in-care' children who may be under the care of social services.

FURTHER READING

Bluestone CD. Paediatric otolaryngology: past present and future. *Arch Otolaryngol Head Neck Surg.* 1995;121:505–8. doi: 10.1001/archotol.1995.01890050005001.

General Medical Council (GMC). 0–18 years: guidance for all doctors. Available at: https://www.gmc-uk.org/ethical-guidance/ethical-guidance-for-doctors/0-18-years (accessed 21 January 2022).

Mitchell RB, Archer SM, Ishman SL. Clinical practice guideline: tonsillectomy in children (update) – Executive summary. *Otolaryngol Head Neck Surg.* 2019;160(2):187–205. doi: 10.1177/0194599818807917.

Safe delivery of paediatric ENT surgery in the UK: a national strategy. A report of a combined working party of the British Association for Paediatric Otolaryngology (BAPO), ENT UK, the Royal College of Anaesthetists (RCoA) and the Association of Paediatric Anaesthetists of Great Britain and Ireland (APAGBI). Available at: https://www.bapo.co.uk/introducing-the-safe-delivery-of-paediatric-ent-surgery-in-the-uk-a-national-strategy/ (accessed 21 January 2022).

2

THE PAEDIATRIC CONSULTATION

INTRODUCTION

Otolaryngologists are well trained in history taking and examination for adults with disorders of the head and neck, but there are aspects of the paediatric consultation that set it apart.

A good first meeting with a child is a unique opportunity for you, the clinician, to establish a rapport with them and their family that may persist well into the child's adult life. The health and welfare of the child are paramount and must be at the forefront of any plans made, but the decision to see you will have typically come from the parents (often the mother) and this makes for some important differences between the adult and paediatric consultation; the diagnosis, the discussion of management options and the decision making are essentially 'by proxy' and they will usually involve the parents or carers rather than the child. The older child may be able to express their views, but with babies and young children, you need to look after essentially two patients, the child and the parent or parents.

HISTORY

Take time to read the case notes, including the results of investigations if applicable, before the child enters the room. Case records are often electronic, and it can be disconcerting for the child and the parent if the doctor is constantly turning to look at their computer screen. Greet the child by name, make eye contact, and introduce yourself and any other staff in the room. Establish who is with the child – it may be a parent, a carer or a grandparent. Be clear on who is going to give you the history and make sure the child is given the opportunity to speak if they are old enough.

The birth history, whether the child needed a stay on a special care baby unit (SCBU), whether the baby needed ET intubation or any form of airway support or had feeding difficulties are especially important considerations in the ORL clinic. If the child has a chronic medical condition or a syndrome, read up on it before you see the family if you can. This should be easy in most settings as so much information is available online. Parent and child will appreciate continuity, and if you are seeing a child for repeat visits, it is ideal if the same doctor sees them each time.

DOI: 10.1201/9780429019128-2

The worldwide COVID-19 pandemic has brought about an increased need for remote consultation – by video link or by telephone – and clinicians have had to develop the skills to take detailed histories in this way (see Chapter 29).

EXAMINATION

Begin your examination as soon as the child comes into the room. Note the child's gait, breathing pattern and state of alertness. Once they have had a little while to settle in the clinic room, most children are happy to be examined. Smaller children are best examined sitting on their mother's knee. It is reasonable for the mother to gently hold the child, but it is not appropriate to restrain a child for a clinical examination; do not persist if they are fractious or struggling. A preliminary nasal examination includes an assessment of the nasal airway, and the 'cold spatula test' (placing a cold stainless-steel instrument with a flat surface under the child's nostrils during quiet breathing to test for condensation). This is especially useful in young children. Children do not like the Thudicum's speculum; get a good view of the nasal cavities by gently elevating the tip of the nose using your thumb and inspecting the nose with a good light source such as a headlight or an otoscope (**Figure 2.1**).

Tongue depressors are not popular with children either; you can usually get a good view of the pharynx using a standard headlight as the child elevates the palate by saying '*Ahhh*'. Endoscopes, both flexible and rigid, are increasingly the norm in ORL clinics and can make for an excellent view of the nose, nasopharynx and laryngeal introitus in co-operative children. It can be especially helpful to project the image onto a large screen so the child and parent can see it.

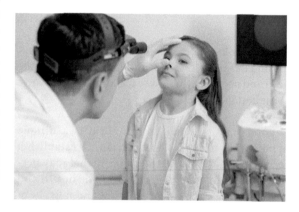

Figure 2.1 Nasal examination. Use a good light source and gently elevate the tip of the nose.

NORMAL GROWTH AND DEVELOPMENT

ORL doctors are not medical paediatricians, but many conditions that are more properly the preserve of paediatricians will present to the ORL clinic. Delayed speech, hearing difficulties and balance disorders may be markers for global developmental delay, autistic spectrum disorders (ASDs) or neurodevelopmental conditions. It is wise to be aware of some of the expected milestones in child growth and development so that you can make appropriate referrals when there is concern. Remember that there is great variation even within families as to how quickly different skills develop. Parents will usually have a careful record of their child's progress, often in the form of an official health record (**Figure 2.2**). The Personal Child Health Record (PCHR, 'red book') in the UK contains a wealth of data which parents can refer to and presents an opportunity for them and their health professionals to fill in details as the child progresses. The 'red book', or its equivalent, can be a very useful source of information during a consultation. Electronic records that can easily be stored on a mobile phone are becoming more common.

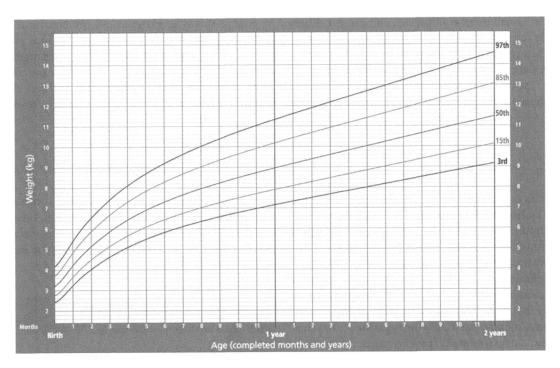

Figure 2.2 Example growth chart from the 'red book': WHO weight-for-age, girls, birth to 2 years (percentiles).

CHILD PROTECTION

Looking after the safety and welfare of children is everybody's responsibility. It is a sad fact that children are sometimes subject to physical, emotional and sexual abuse. This may be perpetrated by family members, friends and acquaintances, or even by professionals who come in contact with children. Regulatory bodies such as the General Medical Council (GMC) in the UK expect doctors to be conversant with the tell-tale signs of abuse or neglect and to act quickly on any concerns they may have. Most hospitals will arrange training for healthcare personnel to make them aware of the path to follow in the event of any concerns, and will usually signpost clinicians to more experienced staff who have specific expertise in these matters. If you find yourself in a situation where you are worried, seek senior help according to the arrangements in place locally. This is an area of great sensitivity. An accusation or suspicion of abuse or neglect can cause great distress if it is unfounded, or prejudice appropriate action if it is

well-founded but not handled with extreme delicacy. Around 75% of children who suffer physical abuse have injuries to the head and neck (**Box 2.1**).

Box 2.1 Possible signs of abuse in ORL

- Tears to the lingual frenulum
- Bruises to the cheeks, lips, gums
- Nasal injuries
- Injuries to the pinna, especially 'pinch' marks
- Auricular haematomas
- Traumatic perforation of the eardrum
- Maxillofacial fractures
- Dental trauma
- Injuries to the palate, e.g. due to forceful feeding
- Bruising to the neck

A very small number of parents and carers deliberately cause or feign symptoms and signs of disease in their children. ORL examples include ear injuries, blocked tracheostomy tubes and deliberate smothering. The term 'Fabricated or Induced Illness (FII)' is preferred to the older term 'Munchausen's syndrome by proxy'. This is an extreme and complex form of child abuse and may be evidence of a serious psychiatric condition in the parent. FII requires urgent, skilled and expert management. If you have any concerns, admit the child for observation and seek the help and advice of an experienced paediatric team.

FUNCTIONAL ORL DISORDERS

Just as in the adult world, children present to the ORL clinic with symptoms for which no organic pathophysiological cause can be found despite a thorough examination and following extensive investigations. The term 'functional disorders' emphasises that although there is no structural or demonstrable anatomical abnormality, there may be very real physiological dysfunction. Terms such as 'medically unexplained', 'psychogenic', 'stress-related', 'psychosomatic' and 'hysterical' were used in the past but are unhelpful and became derogatory with the implication of blame on the part of the patient. These symptoms are very real, cause immense distress and warrant thorough and sensitive investigation and management. ORL symptoms include earache, tinnitus, dysphagia, balance disorders, dysphonia and, very rarely, stridor. Functional or 'non-organic' hearing loss (see Chapter 7) is well recognised. Parental disharmony, bullying – increasingly 'online' – and the physiological and psychological changes of puberty can all have an impact on child health and somatic symptoms often come to the fore. A sensitive and thoughtful explanation of the symptoms, with reassurance that there is no worrying progressive pathology and that the prognosis is good, is often all that is required. The worldwide COVID pandemic has caused a great deal of often unrecognised distress to both adults and children, and somatic manifestations and functional disorders seem to be on the increase. Children do, of course, develop depression, severe life-threatening eating disorders and very rarely psychosis; in such cases, expert psychiatric help will be needed.

KEY POINTS

- Children with neurodevelopmental disorders may present to ORL. If in any doubt, seek a paediatric opinion.
- Child protection and promoting good child health are everybody's business.
- 'Functional' disorders are not the same as feigned or factitious illness. Many are short-lived and should not be 'over-medicalised'.

FURTHER READING

Electronic 'eredbook'. Available at: https://www.eredbook.org.uk (accessed 21 January 2022).

Royal College of Paediatrics and Child Health (RCPCH). Resources and advice on child protection and safeguarding. Available at: https://www.rcpch.ac.uk/key-topics/child-protection (accessed 21 January 2022).

3 CHILDREN WITH SPECIAL NEEDS

INTRODUCTION

All children are special. Some have unique medical or developmental difficulties which create needs in addition to those of their age-matched peers. The term 'special needs' encompasses a huge range including children with mild learning disability, developmental delay, severe motor and sensory neurological impairment, attention deficit hyperactivity disorder (ADHD) and ASDs.

Children in the ORL clinic often have a 'syndrome' or a series of medical issues that constitute a 'sequence' or an 'association'.

SYNDROMES, SEQUENCES AND ASSOCIATIONS

A *syndrome* is a group of birth defects with a single (usually genetic) cause, e.g. *Down syndrome (trisomy 21)*.

In a *sequence*, the clinical features are due to a single anatomical abnormality, e.g. in *Pierre Robin sequence*, it is the hypoplasia of the lower facial skeleton that causes micrognathia, tongue base prolapse and palatal defects.

An *association* is a group of defects that commonly occur together, without a specific known cause, e.g. *VATER, CHARGE* (see below).

Some syndromes, sequences and associations with ORL manifestations are listed in **Box 3.1**.

■ Down syndrome (trisomy 21)

The genetic anomaly in Down syndrome is the presence of an extra chromosome 21, hence the term 'trisomy 21' (**Figure 3.1**). Children with Down syndrome are prone to a variety of ENT pathologies. They have a high incidence of OSA due to muscle hypotonia, relative macroglossia due to a mid-facial hypoplasia, and large obstructing tonsils and adenoids. Congenital heart disease is more prevalent than in age-matched peers, and OSA can precipitate pulmonary hypertension, a serious and potentially devastating feature of trisomy 21. Airway problems are common and include tracheo-oesophageal fistula (TOF), tracheomalacia and subglottic stenosis (SGS). Other ENT issues include deafness, both sensorineural

DOI: 10.1201/9780429019128-3

Box 3.1 Some syndromes, sequences and associations with ORL manifestations

Syndromes

- Down syndrome (trisomy 21)
- Turner's syndrome
- Treacher Collins syndrome
- Goldenhar's syndrome
- Crouzon's syndrome
- Apert's syndrome
- 22Q11 deletion syndrome
- CHARGE syndrome
- Syndromes causing congenital deafness

Sequences and associations

- Pierre Robin sequence
- VATER association
- CHARGE association

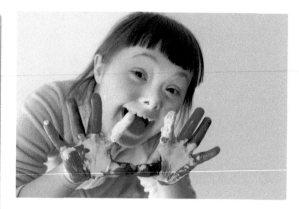

Figure 3.1 A girl with Down syndrome (trisomy 21).

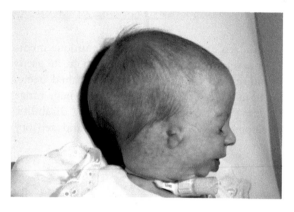

Figure 3.2 A baby with Treacher Collins syndrome. Note she has microtia and micrognathia. Tracheotomy was performed soon after birth.

and conductive. A small external ear canal, a high incidence of otitis media with effusion (OME) and anatomical abnormalities of the ossicles, cochlea and facial nerve are all well documented. Thyroid pathology is also more common.

Children with Down syndrome often feature on ENT operating lists and the surgeon and anaesthetist need to be aware of some particular issues relating to perioperative care. For example, a child with Down syndrome will often need a smaller-sized ET tube than their age-matched peer and have a tendency for atlantoaxial instability, so the child's head has to be manipulated with special care.

▌ Turner's syndrome

Girls with this syndrome have the sex chromosome make-up XO. ENT issues are common and include both sensorineural deafness and conductive deafness, a high incidence of cleft palate and abnormalities of the pinna.

▌ Treacher Collins syndrome

This is now known to be caused by a gene defect, most commonly in the *TOCF1* gene which codes for a protein known as 'treacle'. It is inherited in an autosomal dominant pattern but with varying severity. ENT features include abnormalities of the pinna, microtia, conductive deafness, cleft palate, choanal atresia, and mandibular and maxillary hypoplasia. Micrognathia can cause severe airway problems necessitating a tracheostomy (**Figure 3.2**).

Craniofacial syndromes

Conditions such as *Goldenhar's, Crouzon's, Pfeiffer's* and *Apert's syndromes* are characterised by craniofacial dysmorphism, often with hemifacial microsomia, craniosynostosis (premature fusion of the skull sutures), microtia, mandibular and maxillary hypoplasia, cleft palate and often severe airway problems needing tracheostomy.

Sensorineural hearing loss

A number of specific syndromes (e.g. *Waardenburg's, Pendred's, Alport's* and *Jervel/Lange Neilson syndrome*) are known causes of profound sensorineural hearing loss and are seen in cochlear implant clinics.

22Q11 deletion syndrome (formerly known as DiGeorge syndrome) is increasingly recognised as a cause of sensorineural deafness.

Pierre Robin sequence

This is characterised by mandibular hypoplasia, cleft palate and micrognathia. Glossoptosis – a tendency of the tongue to prolapse back into the airway – contributes to airway obstruction. Feeding problems are common and these babies are best nursed prone in contrast with the usual advice to put babies on their backs – *'back to sleep'*. They may need a nasopharyngeal airway but the airway improves as the baby develops and the mandible grows. Nowadays, tracheostomy is very rarely needed.

VATER (VACTERL) association

This association, characterised by **v**ertebral, **a**norectal, **c**ardiac, **t**racheal, **e**sophageal, **r**enal and **l**imb abnormalities, is not uncommon in paediatric practice and some of these babies may also have ENT conditions as well (e.g. tracheomalacia, SGS).

CHARGE

CHARGE is characterised by **c**oloboma (an ocular anomaly), **h**eart defects, **a**tresia of the choanae, **g**rowth defects (often genital hypoplasia), **r**enal abnormalities and **e**ar defects. ENT surgeons often diagnose the condition as it presents with severe airway obstruction in the newborn due to choanal atresia (see Chapter 22). CHARGE is now regarded as in some cases a syndrome rather than an association, as a range of specific genetic causes have been identified, notably a mutation of gene *CHD7*.

NEURODEVELOPMENTAL CONDITIONS

ORL specialists are seeing children in increasing numbers with ASD. This is a complex and, as yet, incompletely understood spectrum of developmental conditions characterised by impaired social interaction and communication, often with repetitive behaviour patterns. It varies greatly in severity and is especially important in ORL as children may present with language delay and the diagnosis is often delayed. The reason for the greatly increased prevalence is unclear, but greater awareness and wider diagnostic criteria are probably important. Children with ASD need particularly sensitive management if they are scheduled for surgery as some may find the company of other children distressing and may become very upset if they have to wait for long periods. There is no 'typical' pattern with ASD and each child has different features, needs and responses. Close liaison with the anaesthetist, ward staff and theatre staff but *especially the parents* to plan admission and discharge will make for a much happier experience for all.

ADHD is an umbrella term used to describe a series of behavioural conditions associated with hyperactivity, impulsiveness, a poor attention span and often disruptive behaviour. Suspected or actual hearing loss and poor sleep patterns can be reasons for presentation to ORL. ASD and ADHD are very different

KEY POINTS

- One of the paradoxes of looking after children is that, despite their smaller size, they require more clinic space than adults. This is especially true in children with special needs.
- ADHD is characterised by hyperactivity, impulsivity and inattention, but many children will exhibit these characteristics in varying degrees.
- Children with ASD may present to the ORL clinic with delayed speech and apparent hearing loss.
- Be sensitive with your language when dealing with the parents of children with syndromes. Refer to the child first and the condition later. Parents prefer the term 'a child with Down syndrome' to 'a Down syndrome child'. When comparing the progress of a child with a syndrome to another child, avoid the use of terms such as 'normal'. A child with Down syndrome, for example, is more likely to have middle ear effusions than a 'typically developing child' rather than a 'normal' child. Attention to such subtleties makes for a far better rapport with parents.
- Children with syndromes usually need intensive multidisciplinary input but are increasingly seen in ENT clinics. Many will have cochlear implants (CIs), bone-anchored hearing aids (BAHAs) and tracheostomies.
- Parents are usually very familiar with the features of their child's syndrome and may be members of one of a number of patient/parent support groups.

conditions but they may coexist, and children suspected of either will need referral to the appropriate paediatric or psychology team for skilled assessment and diagnosis.

FURTHER READING

British Association for Paediatric Otolaryngology (BAPO). Available at: https://www.bapo.co.uk/ (accessed 21 January 2022).

Chin CJ, Khami MM, Husein M. A general review of the otolaryngologic manifestations of Down Syndrome. *Int J Pediatr Otorhinolaryngol.* 2014; 78(6):899–904. doi: 10.1016/j.ijporl.2014.03.012.

Down's Syndrome Association (DSA). Available at: http://www.downs-syndrome.org.uk/for-new-parents/ (accessed 21 January 2022).

National Organization for Rare Disorders (NORD). Available at: https://rarediseases.org (accessed 21 January 2022).

4 ENT FOREIGN BODIES

INTRODUCTION

Children are curious. They like to explore and experiment, often putting objects in places they shouldn't – including in their ears, noses and throats. If they don't do this themselves, a sibling or school or nursery friend may. The child will not always volunteer or admit what has happened, hence the need for vigilance when there is any suspicion.

EAR

Toys, pieces of crayon, beads, sponge, organic matter such as food particles and even live insects can be found in the ear canal. The parent or carer may witness the child putting something in their ear, or an object can be found incidentally on otoscopy. Often, there is no pain or discharge, but organic matter can become infected. Wax tends to accumulate around the object and may become impacted. Gentle suction under vision (microscopy) or syringing with warm water may be enough, but if the object is impacted, or very deep in the ear canal, it will need instrumental removal. Use a 'grasping' instrument, 'crocodile' or 'alligator' forceps, under good lighting conditions and with the child relaxed and quiet if the object has an irregular edge. A spherical object (e.g. a bead) is better removed using a curved or hooked instrument introduced to be able to get behind the object and gently withdraw it. If the child is fractious or very nervous, you may need to arrange a general anaesthetic. Live insects can cause intense distress; immobilise the insect by filling the ear canal with a local anaesthetic (lidocaine) prior to removal.

NOSE

Nasal foreign bodies often pass into the pharynx and are harmlessly swallowed. Impacted objects include crayons, chalk, beads, sponge and small toys. Presentation can be early if the parent or carer sees the event or the child admits it, but often the object stays impacted in the nose for days or weeks until it causes infection, a discharge (sometimes foul-smelling), with bleeding and excoriation of the skin

DOI: 10.1201/9780429019128-4

around the nostril (**Figure 4.1**). Remove the object if you can in the outpatient setting using a good light and suitable instrument. A hooked or curved instrument is best, otherwise the object may be pushed further back. A fractious or nervous child, especially if the object has been in for some time and has become crusted and adherent, will need a general anaesthetic. This is best arranged soon, ideally within a day or so of seeing the child. If the child is otherwise well and has no neurological issues (i.e. has a good swallow and no tendency to aspiration), the risk of inhalation is extremely low.

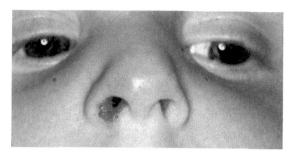

Figure 4.1 Excoriation of the skin around the nostril caused by a retained nasal foreign body.

INGESTED FOREIGN BODIES

Coins, toys and small household objects including most dangerously 'button batteries' are easily swallowed especially by toddlers who are inclined to explore and very often put objects into their mouths. Many are innocuous and pass into the stomach and beyond with no ill-effects, but some may impact at the level of the vallecula, cricopharyngeus or mid-oesophagus. There may be a definite history, and the child will complain of difficulty with swallowing, but presentation can be delayed. Some objects such as a food bolus or a large coin can compress the trachea and cause acute airway obstruction. A sharp object, a pin or nail, can cause oesophageal perforation. An impacted pharyngeal or oesophageal foreign body will need to be removed under general anaesthesia, ideally within a few hours. Button batteries are especially destructive, with the capacity to erode the oesophageal mucosa and cause catastrophic bleeding in the mediastinal great vessels so need immediate removal, even if the child has a full stomach.

INHALED FOREIGN BODIES

Babies and toddlers may inhale various objects they put in their mouths, sometimes with devastating consequences. The event is not always witnessed, and coughing, choking, shortness of breath and sudden onset of stridor or 'wheezing' may be the first signs something is amiss. An object impacted in the larynx or trachea can be fatal. Immediate first-aid measures at the time (e.g. a series of sharp blows to the supine baby's back or in an older child a 'Heimlich' manoeuvre) can be lifesaving.

A foreign body that passes into the bronchus will cause some degree of oxygen desaturation, but the child will usually breathe well using the other lung. Not all foreign bodies are radiopaque, but a chest X-ray is nevertheless helpful and may

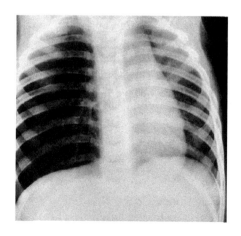

Figure 4.2 Chest X-ray showing obstructive emphysema.

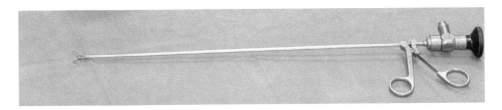

Figure 4.3 Optical forceps for removal of a bronchial foreign body.

show hyperinflation of the lung on the side of the obstruction due to reduced airflow in expiration ('obstructive emphysema', **Figure 4.2**). If there is reasonable suspicion of a bronchial foreign body, arrange airway endoscopy (tracheobronchoscopy) quickly, but with care to ensure that the surgeon, anaesthetist and nursing team have the appropriate experience and equipment including ventilating bronchoscopes, a series of optical 'grasping' forceps (**Figure 4.3**) and postoperative recovery and care facilities. Organic objects, such as peanuts and food particles, cause a local inflammatory reaction and, if any foreign body has been present for a prolonged period, recovery may be complicated by the development of long-term bronchopulmonary disease (bronchiectasis).

CAUSTIC INJURIES

Caustic agents such as detergents, bleach, oven-cleaning fluid and various household cleaning substances may be ingested by toddlers. Devastating injuries to the mouth, pharynx, larynx and oesophagus can result. Public health measures such as safer containers and increased awareness of the dangers have greatly reduced the incidence, but tragic accidents still occur. If caustic ingestion is suspected, admit the child urgently and consider early and careful endoscopy. Complications include oesophageal stenosis, laryngotracheal cicatrisation and scarring of the tissues of the mouth and pharynx, sometimes requiring gastrostomy feeding and long-term tracheostomy.

BUTTON BATTERIES

'Button batteries' are ubiquitous now in household electronic devices, hearing aids and some toys (**Figure 4.4**). They are extremely powerful and can be quickly destructive if they come in contact with tissues. In the ear canal, they may cause intense inflammation with bone erosion and they can cause septal perforation and long-term stenosis in the nose. A battery is especially destructive if swallowed when it may impact at the cricopharyngeus or mid-oesophagus and erode through the lumen. Fatal mediastinal bleeds have been reported, and prolonged oesophageal stenosis is not uncommon. The destructive effects can be delayed and occur long after the battery has been removed.

If you suspect a child has ingested a button battery, make immediate arrangements to get them to an operating theatre for pharyngo-oesophagoscopy and removal. There is some evidence that oral administration of honey may be a helpful first-aid measure. The degree of urgency is such that the child should have a general anaesthetic even with a full stomach, as the balance of risk of tissue destruction from the battery versus the hazards of possible aspiration of stomach contents is such as to warrant immediate endoscopy.

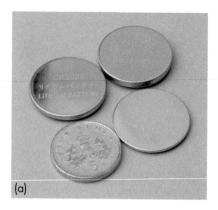
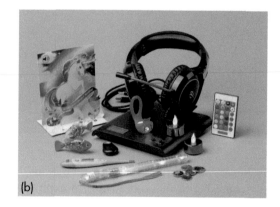

Figure 4.4 (a) Button batteries (coin shown to illustrate size) and (b) some common household items that require button batteries.

KEY POINTS

- Don't persist in the emergency department (ED) trying to remove a nasal or ear foreign body if the child is fractious or distressed. Refer to the ENT clinic or arrange a general anaesthetic.
- Modern 'button batteries' are very powerful and can cause severe destruction of tissues. If you suspect a child has ingested or inhaled a button battery, get the child to an operating theatre for removal of the battery without delay – even if the child has a full stomach.

FURTHER READING

Houston R, Powell S, Jaffray B, Ball S. Clinical guideline for retained button batteries. *Arch Dis Child*. 2021;106(2):192–4. doi: 10.1136/archdischild-2019-318354.

Shaffer AD, Jacobs IN, Derkay CS et al. Management and outcomes of button batteries in the aerodigestive tract: a multi-institutional study. *Laryngoscope*. 2021;131(1):E298–E306. doi: 10.1002/lary.28568.

5
SEPSIS IN THE HEAD AND NECK

INTRODUCTION

The ears, nose and throat are the entry portals to the upper respiratory tract and are subject to a range of infections which can spread to adjacent areas – notably the fascial spaces of the neck, the periorbital tissues and the mastoid air cells. Intracranial sepsis and fulminant mediastinitis may be secondary to an infection that started in the upper respiratory tract, and haematogenous spread of pyogenic organisms can cause devastating systemic sepsis.

DEEP NECK SPACE INFECTIONS

The fascial layers of the neck – the superficial and deep cervical fascia – are distributed so as to create a number of potential spaces where abscesses can collect and expand (**Figures 5.1** and **5.2**) and deep neck space (DNS) infections can develop. Infection in the oropharynx, especially the tonsil, can easily spread to cause suppuration in the parapharyngeal space, the peritonsillar space or, in very young children, the retropharyngeal lymph nodes. Dental infections can spread to the submental and submandibular space. The flora are mainly the pyogenic (pus-producing) organisms – *Streptococcus pneumoniae*, *Staphylococcus aureus* and *Haemophilus influenzae* – but anaerobes and unusual organisms may be implicated.

An abscess in the parapharyngeal space produces a tense, painful swelling in the side of the neck in a febrile child, with erythema and cellulitis of the skin. Admit the child, commence IV hydration, antibiotics,

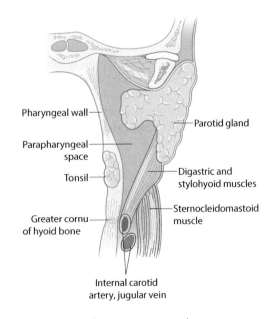

Pharyngeal wall

Parapharyngeal space

Tonsil

Greater cornu of hyoid bone

Parotid gland

Digastric and stylohyoid muscles

Sternocleidomastoid muscle

Internal carotid artery, jugular vein

Figure 5.1 Neck spaces – coronal view.

DOI: 10.1201/9780429019128-5

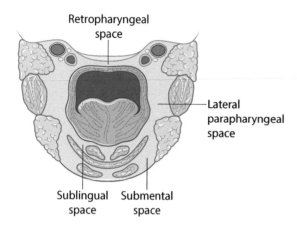

Figure 5.2 Neck spaces – lateral view.

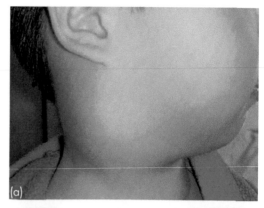

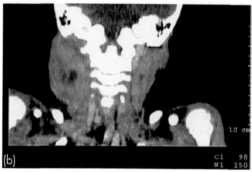

Figure 5.3 (a,b) Parapharyngeal abscess. The abscess has become organised (phlegmon).

analgesia as required and measure baseline observations. If the child is especially toxic or there is no early response to antimicrobial therapy, arrange for incision and drainage under general anaesthetic. The abscess is fluctuant in the early stages and incision and drainage are likely to allow pus to escape, but the abscess may have become firm and indurated and organised such that there is little or no pus (a *phlegmon*). Ultrasound scanning can help by showing the fluid. A computed tomography (CT) scan may be helpful especially if it can be undertaken without a general anaesthetic (**Figure 5.3**).

A *retropharyngeal abscess* occurs typically in younger children (up to the age of about 3 years) who tend to have prominent lymph nodes in the retropharyngeal space. The child will flex their neck and extend the head; dysphagia or a painful swallow causes drooling. Stertorous breathing suggests some degree of airway obstruction, and the child is at risk of asphyxia.

Treatment is initially with systemic antibiotics, progressing to incision and drainage if there is no rapid resolution. Anaesthesia in these children can be difficult as the pharyngeal swelling makes ET intubation especially challenging. They often need to be transferred to a specialist paediatric unit for transoral incision and drainage (**Figure 5.4**).

Peritonsillar abscess (quinsy) is mainly a condition of older children and young adults. If treated early,

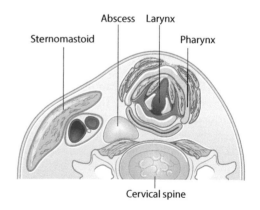

Figure 5.4 Retropharyngeal abscess.

antimicrobial therapy may suffice, but a large abscess will require incision and drainage. Some surgeons advocate 'quinsy tonsillectomy' – a 'hot' tonsillectomy – particularly if the child would need a general anaesthetic for incision and drainage.

Suppuration in the floor of the mouth can complicate a dental infection. Incision and drainage may be very unrewarding as there is extensive cellulitis with induration of the tissues (*Ludwig's angina*).

DNS infections usually resolve with a good outcome, but infection may spread to the mediastinum, along the carotid sheath, and to the intracranial structures. Haematogenous spread can give rise to septicaemia with devastating consequences.

MASTOID ABSCESS

Acute otitis media (AOM) invariably involves some degree of inflammatory changes in the mucosa of the mastoid air cells. Redness of the skin and a fluctuant swelling of the tissues over the mastoid process (**Figure 5.5**) suggest that the infection has escaped the bony confines of the temporal bone and formed a sub-periosteal abscess which, if unchecked, will rupture through the periosteum, involve the venous sinuses (venous sinus thrombosis) and extend beyond the dura potentially to cause serious neurological complications.

Intense IV antimicrobial therapy may suffice in the early stages, but a fluctuant abscess may need drainage, to include a cortical mastoidectomy and an extensive myringotomy to allow pus to escape from the middle ear. The diagnosis is clinical but a CT scan may delineate the extent of the abscess and help with surgical planning.

Gradenigo's triad/syndrome – VI nerve palsy, pain in the distribution of the trigeminal nerve and otitis

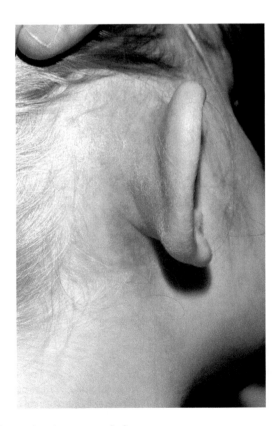

Figure 5.5 Acute mastoiditis with sub-periosteal abscess.

media – occurs when an abscess forms in the petrous apex. *Bezold's abscess* is a collection of pus in the neck due to tracking of infection behind the sternomastoid. *Lemierre's syndrome* is a septic thrombosis of the internal jugular vein, usually secondary to mastoiditis due to the bacterium *Fusobacterium necrophorum*.

ORBITAL CELLULITIS

Paranasal sinus infections can be complicated by spread beyond the bony confines of the sinuses. Frontal sinus abscess (*Pott's puffy tumour*) is now very rare. Sinogenic intracranial abscess is uncommon but orbital sepsis is still a frequent mode of presentation of children with sinus infection. Infection easily breaks through the thin party wall between the ethmoid sinuses and the orbit (the lamina papyracea). Swelling and erythema of the soft tissues of the orbit (orbital cellulitis) ensue and may progress to abscess formation with proptosis requiring urgent decompression (incision and drainage usually via an external approach at the medial canthus) or even, in extreme cases, to cavernous sinus thrombosis with ophthalmoplegia and a serious risk to vision. Admit the child, commence IV hydration, antibiotics, and consider surgery if there is an abscess.

INTRACRANIAL COMPLICATIONS

Otitis media, mastoiditis and sinusitis can be complicated by spread of infection beyond the dura (**Figures 5.6–5.8**). Severe headache, pain out of proportion to the otoscopic findings, extreme systemic toxicity and, most of all, alteration in consciousness or focal neurological signs should raise suspicion. Imaging is especially helpful here. The child with suspected intracranial sepsis needs urgent admission, antimicrobial therapy and neurosurgical review.

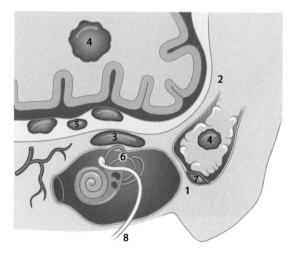

Figure 5.6 Some potential complications of otitis media: 1. Mastoiditis; 2. Petrous apex abscess; 3. Extradural abscess; 4. Intracranial abscess – cerebral or cerebellar; 5. Subdural abscess; 6. Labyrinthitis; 7. Venous sinus thrombosis; 8. Facial palsy.

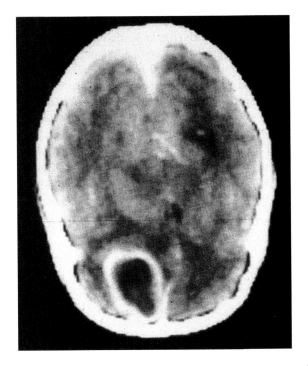

Figure 5.7 Frontal lobe sinogenic abscess.

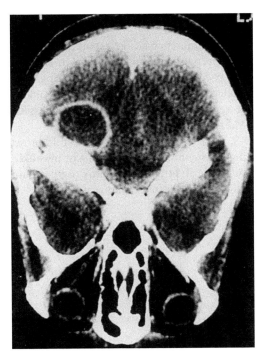

Figure 5.8 CT scan showing otogenic intracranial abscess.

SYSTEMIC SEPSIS

There is increasing recognition that children can develop a life-threatening, rapidly progressive exaggerated inflammatory response to infection. This has come to be known as 'sepsis' and is a time-critical emergency that warrants immediate intervention. Children can deteriorate alarmingly quickly, and an apparently healthy baby with what initially seems a mild respiratory infection may become moribund in a short period. If you have any worries regarding a child's worsening condition, be mindful of the local arrangements with regard to paediatric early warning signs (PEWS), monitor the child's condition carefully and commence antimicrobial and fluid replacement therapy immediately, ideally in consultation with an experienced paediatric team.

KEY POINTS

- The ears, nose and throat are the entry portals to the upper respiratory tract and are subject to a range of infections which can spread to adjacent areas.
- Sepsis is a time-critical emergency. Children can deteriorate very quickly.

FURTHER READING

https://qicentral.rcpch.ac.uk/resources/systems-of-care/recognition-and-response-to-sepsis-in-the-paediatric-emergency-care-setting/ Royal College Paediatrics and Child HealthGuidelines re sepsis in children, May 2020 (accessed 29 March 2022).

Patel S, Burgess A. Guideline for the child presenting to hospital with otitis media or mastoiditis. Available at: https://www.entuk.org/paediatric-guidelines (accessed 21 January 2022).

Patel S, Burgess A. Guideline for the child presenting to hospital with lymphadenitis or a lymph node abscess. Available at: www.entuk.org/paediatric-guidelines (accessed 21 January 2022).

Patel S, Burgess A. Guideline for the child presenting to hospital with tonsillitis or quinsy. Available at: www.entuk.org/paediatric-guidelines (accessed 21 January 2022).

Patel S, Burgess A, Marsh C. Guideline for the child presenting to hospital with pre-septal or post-septal cellulitis. Available at: www.entuk.org/paediatric-guidelines (accessed 21 January 2022).

6
THE EXTERNAL EAR

DEVELOPMENT OF THE EAR

The external ear includes the pinna and the external ear canal. The pinna and the outer part of the ear canal are made of cartilage, covered by perichondrium and skin. A series of 'hillocks' derived from the first two branchial (pharyngeal) arches fuse to become the external ear, and developmental abnormalities are fairly common.

CONGENITAL ANOMALIES

■ 'Minor' anomalies

These include skin tags, pre-auricular sinuses, appendages, cysts and 'accessory auricles'. They can be upsetting for parents but can usually be treated surgically if they give rise to aesthetic concerns or recurrent infection. A 'pre-auricular sinus' is a small blind-ending pit, lined with squamous epithelium and lying just in front of the pinna. This is usually innocuous but can become infected; it is easily removed by wide local excision, ideally when the child is about 2 years old (**Figure 6.1**). A 'pre-auricular sinus' is not to be confused with a branchial or 'first arch' abnormality, which is usually lower (below the tragus), and can be a marker for a complex tract (fistula) running into the ear canal (see Chapter 26). Some congenital abnormalities, including the not-uncommon 'accessory auricle', are shown in **Figure 6.2**.

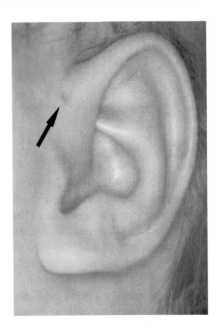

Figure 6.1 Pre-auricular sinus.

DOI: 10.1201/9780429019128-6

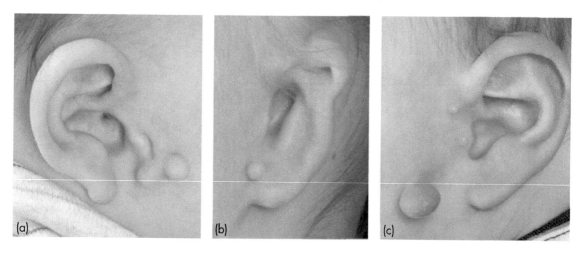

Figure 6.2 Congenital external ear abnormalities: (a) Deformity of the pinna with accessory auricle; (b) accessory auricle with microtia (c) accessory auricle with normal pinna.

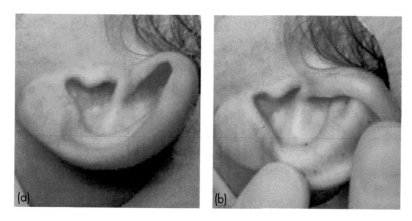

Figure 6.3 (a,b) Prominent ear with poorly developed anti-helical fold.

▌▌ Prominent ears

'Protruding ears' (often unkindly referred to as 'bat ears') are a common reason for referral of a child to an otolaryngology or plastic surgery clinic. The child is often subject to bullying and name-calling and may become very distressed. The typical deformity is a poorly developed or absent anti-helical fold (**Figure 6.3**). If the parents of a newborn baby present, some degree of moulding of the cartilage can be brought about by the use of specially designed splints (EarBuddies™, **Figure 6.4**) but, in older children, the treatment is surgical. Most authorities regard the age

of about 4 to 5 years as ideal, before the child is settled in school. There are multiple surgical techniques to re-contour the anti-helical fold. Careful preoperative planning, including clinical photography and detailed counselling of the parents regarding the expectations of surgery, is important.

▌▌ Microtia

More serious abnormalities of development range from *microtia* (literally a 'small ear') to *anotia*, which is absence of all of the structures that make up the external ear (**Figure 6.5**).

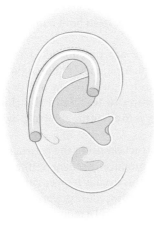

Figure 6.4 Splint to correct prominent ear.

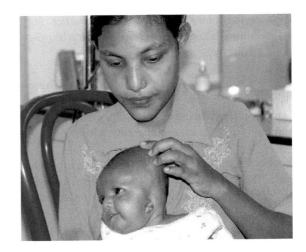

Figure 6.5 Baby with high-grade microtia

Microtia can be unilateral (far more common, 4 : 1) or bilateral, and has a prevalence of 2.5 in 10 000 births. In addition to the external ear deformity, there may be canal atresia or stenosis. There can be associated ossicular, middle ear and inner ear abnormalities. The issues are both aesthetic and functional; associated hearing loss is common but not universal.

In the majority of cases, microtia presents as an isolated deformity in an otherwise healthy child, but it can be part of a spectrum of abnormalities in syndromes such as *branchio-oto-renal syndrome*, *hemifacial microsomia*, *Goldenhar syndrome* and *Treacher Collins syndrome*. Maternal rubella infection – now uncommon due to widespread vaccination – has been considered a factor in microtia. Some drugs in pregnancy such as thalidomide (no longer used) and isotretinoin (sometimes given for acne) have also been implicated, but the aetiology is usually unknown.

When a surgeon first meets a baby with microtia, they will need to consider a long and hopefully rewarding relationship with the patient and family. Surgical expertise is best offered in a team that should be able to provide audiological assessment and rehabilitation as well as psychological support throughout the patient's journey. Although there is sometimes a strong parental desire to expedite surgery, the decision should be patient-led with as much information and support provided to help with the decision making. Surgery is often best delayed until the patient is old enough to contribute to the decision-making process, which will affect the child for the rest of their life.

Immediate management should focus on optimising hearing. Babies with microtia need a detailed and skilled hearing assessment within the first few weeks of life. Both air and bone conduction thresholds should be determined, and a plan can then be made for early audiological rehabilitation if needed.

In microtia with canal atresia, there is usually a severe conductive hearing loss on the affected side. Inner ear function tends to be good, resulting in some ability to hear on the affected side. The hearing in the contralateral ear is usually normal and, if so, parents can be reassured that speech and language development should progress well. If there is bilateral conductive loss, the baby can be fitted with bone-conducting hearing aids straight away. The Softband® (see Chapter 12, **Figure 12.3**) has proven popular and successful for use with younger children and babies. The child can then be considered for bone-anchored hearing aids (BAHAs) when they are a little older.

The baby should have a full medical paediatric assessment to include whatever investigations are deemed appropriate to look for associated anomalies, (e.g. an abdominal ultrasound to screen for brachio-oto-renal syndrome).

Imaging (CT scan with or without magnetic resonance imaging, MRI) can be left to a later date but can give important information regarding the structure of the middle ear and the inner ear.

The Softband is also used in children with unilateral microtia as the benefits of intervention in single-sided hearing loss are increasingly acknowledged.

The child with microtia is at increased risk of middle ear disease including cholesteatoma, which can be difficult to pick up by otoscopy if there is canal stenosis. Imaging then becomes increasingly important, and the child should have regular audiological and otological surveillance.

A child with microtia presents to the ENT surgeon within the first few weeks or months of life, but a decision with regards to *definitive surgical correction* is best left for several years. Parents will be anxious and will need careful counselling and support, including a full early discussion with a team experienced in the management of this condition and what the possibilities are. The default option – and by far the best approach in the first few years – is simply to observe, and plan intervention as needed when the child is much older.

The aesthetic deformity can be addressed by reconstructive surgery, often using autologous graft material, or a prosthetic implant. It is best if the child

participates fully in the decision as to which route to take, with guidance from both clinician and parent.

Although there are psychological issues for the patient with microtia, most children do not seem to be unduly affected until the age of 6 or 7. The other important reason to wait until the child is older before surgery is to allow the child to grow physically.

Pinna reconstruction using the patient's own costal cartilage can produce excellent aesthetic results in skilled hands. This usually happens at around 9 or 10 years of age. It is a procedure performed in at least two stages scheduled around 6 months apart. The alternative approach is to use a *prosthesis*, using percutaneous abutments to anchor the prosthesis to the skull.

Modern prostheses, fashioned by a skilled technician and customised to the child and the defect, will give a realistic-looking pinna that exactly matches the opposite side. The prosthesis has a fixed lifespan and needs to be changed every 2 years. In addition, as the skin–implant interface is prone to irritation, the patient and family are committed to daily lifelong care of the implant site.

Correction of canal atresia and middle ear surgery for microtia are both highly specialised and technically demanding. The aim is to achieve good hearing, but the serious potential complications of such surgery include facial paralysis, sensorineural hearing loss, and a re-stenosis requiring further surgery. With the excellent hearing results achieved by a BAHA – and the increasingly better BAHAs becoming available – corrective surgery is now rarely indicated.

ACQUIRED PATHOLOGY

▮ Inflammation

Skin disease such as eczema and psoriasis may manifest as otitis externa.

Impacted cerumen can be problematic in children, often made worse by enthusiastic parents who poke objects in the ear in an attempt to remove the wax.

Syringing or gentle suction is usually effective in a cooperative child, and hard wax can be softened by the use of warm olive oil drops for a week or so. True otitis externa is far less common in children than in adults. It can occur following contamination with water – particularly chlorinated or infected water (*swimmer's ear*) – requiring regular suction and the use of local antimicrobial and steroid preparations to

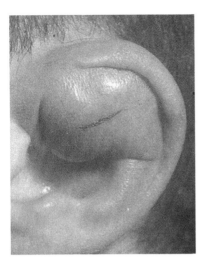

Figure 6.6 Haematoma of the pinna.

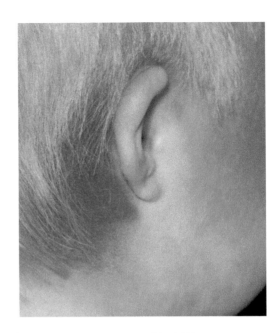

Figure 6.7 Bruising caused by NAI.

keep it under control. An acute staphylococcal infection may produce a tense inflammatory swelling (*furuncle*) as in adults. A streptococcal infection can spread to the pinna to cause a painful erythematous swelling (*erysipelas*). Infection along the tissue planes of the cartilage (*perichondritis*) can, if unchecked, give rise to fibrosis and deformity.

▌ Trauma

Blunt trauma

Blunt trauma to the pinna may cause subcutaneous bleeding leading to a haematoma (**Figure 6.6**). Untreated, this can become infected with scarring and deformity. Consider early evacuation and application of a pressure dressing. A haematoma may be the result of an injury sustained during sport or the 'rough and tumble' of the children's playground but be alert to the possibility of non-accidental injury (NAI). 'Pinchmarks' on the rim of the pinna are said to be pathognomonic of NAI and are caused by rough pinching of the pinna between the finger and thumb when an adult grasps the child by the ear (**Figure 6.7**).

Penetrating trauma

Penetrating trauma is uncommon. Complications of ear-piercing are sometimes seen such as embedded studs, infection, and tears to the lobule if earrings are forcibly removed.

KEY POINTS

- Prominence of the pinna ('bat ears') can cause a great deal of distress to parents and children.
- Improved prostheses have transformed the management of microtia.
- Reconstructive surgery for microtia is best deferred until the child is old enough to make the decision.

FURTHER READING

UK care standards for the management of patients with microtia and atresia. Available at: http://www.bapras.org.uk/docs/default-source/commissioning-and-policy/microtia-and-atresia--care-standards.pdf?sfvrsn=2 (accessed 24 January 2022).

7 HEARING LOSS IN CHILDHOOD

INTRODUCTION

Childhood deafness may be sensorineural, conductive, or mixed and includes auditory neuropathy and auditory processing disorders.

Permanent childhood hearing impairment hearing (PCHI) can be congenital or acquired. It can remain stable, deteriorate progressively, fluctuate or manifest later in life. Conductive loss due to middle ear pathology tends to present later, and it is usually due to acquired childhood pathologies, mainly OME and chronic suppurative otitis media (CSOM) (see Chapters 9 and 11).

Despite improved screening and awareness of the importance of early detection and rehabilitation, which have brought about greatly improved outcomes, deafness in childhood remains a huge global challenge.

INCIDENCE

Between one and two newborn children per thousand are born 'deaf', i.e. with a bilateral permanent childhood hearing impairment (BPCHI). This is usually defined as a hearing loss (HL) of at least 40 dB HL in the better hearing ear. About one-quarter of these children will have 'profound' hearing loss (see Chapter 8) and up to one-third will have significant associated medical issues such as developmental delay or learning difficulties. These figures are even higher in the developing world, where diagnosis is often late and rehabilitation opportunities limited. Screening will detect the great majority of babies with congenital deafness, but delayed-onset hearing loss, often caused by conditions present at or before birth (e.g. intrauterine cytomegalovirus), is well recognised, hence the need for ongoing surveillance for children considered 'at risk'.

AETIOLOGY

The question 'why is my baby deaf' is of great concern to parents. Deafness is a manifestation of one or more pathological processes rather than a final diagnosis, and it is important – but not always possible – to determine an exact aetiology. This helps to outline prognosis and may facilitate specific

DOI: 10.1201/9780429019128-7

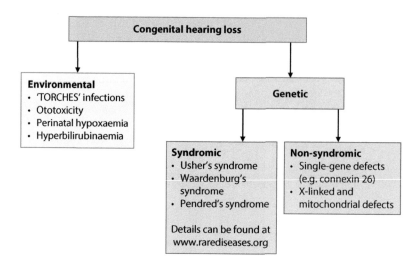

Figure 7.1 Causes of congenital hearing loss.

treatment strategies e.g. antiviral medication in some limited circumstances, and perhaps precise genetic interventions in the future. A definitive diagnosis may also enable referral to appropriate specialists e.g. endocrinologists for Pendred's syndrome, and genetic counselling services.

Congenital (present at birth) hearing loss is traditionally divided into *genetic* (or inherited) causes – more often than not nowadays with a known chromosomal or gene abnormality – and *environmental* causes such as prenatal maternal infection or birth complications such as prolonged hypoxaemia (**Figure 7.1**). Overall, about 50% of cases of congenital deafness are genetically inherited. About another 25% are due to a non-genetic, environmental or acquired pathology.

In about one-third of the inherited or genetic cases, the hearing loss is one manifestation of a 'syndrome' (see Chapter 3), known as *syndromic hearing loss* (see Chapter 8). Most of the remainder are due to recessive genes, a small number are due to dominant genes, and a very small number are due to X-linked or mitochondrial defects. Non-syndromic genetic causes of deafness are highly variable, with different and often unpredictable inheritance patterns.

The specific genetic defect is not always established, but improved detection techniques and gene sequencing are leading to the regular reporting of

new gene mutations causing non-syndromic deafness. Mutations in the gene that codes for connexin 26 – a gap junction protein – are a particularly common finding in permanent congenital hearing impairment (PCHI).

The maternal infections that may be associated with PCHI are often referred to by the acronym TORCHES (**T**oxoplasmosis, **O**ther, **R**ubella, **C**ytomegalovirus, and **H**erpes **S**implex). Toxoplasmosis and rubella are now rare in the developed world, but cytomegalovirus (CMV) in pregnancy is not at all uncommon and about one in a hundred newborns will have some evidence of CMV infection. Only a small number of these (about 5%) will have PCHI but, as the hearing loss may not manifest for the first few weeks, these cases may be missed by newborn screening protocols and babies with CMV should be referred for full audiological evaluation and surveillance. CMV is now the commonest intrauterine infection in humans, and up to 80% of women of reproductive age are seropositive. Some 25% of cases of congenital hearing loss are now associated with CMV infection. Polymerase chain reaction (PCR) testing of the baby's saliva or urine in the first 3 weeks of life will confirm the diagnosis of congenital infection. There is some evidence to support the use of antiviral agents (valgonociclovir) for congenital CMV but only in children with disseminated infection. Trials of antiviral therapy for CMV-associated hearing loss are ongoing.

SCREENING AND SURVEILLANCE

Screening is the testing of individuals among an apparently disease-free population to identify those who warrant further investigation to diagnose a specific condition, in this case PCHI. *Surveillance* for hearing loss is focused on ongoing regular testing and support to include children who may have 'passed' the newborn screen but are still at risk of later-onset PCHI. Some of the conditions that warrant surveillance include babies 'at risk' due to conditions such as extreme prematurity, very low birth weight, severe hyperbilirubinaemia, maternal TORCH infection, ototoxic medication and meningitis.

Most western healthcare systems have introduced 'universal' newborn screening (i.e. of every newborn baby regardless of risk factors), typically by measuring otoacoustic emissions (OAEs, **Figure 7.2**). These are measurable acoustic responses generated in the outer hair cells. The test is easy to perform and relies on inserting an ear tip with a microphone and a speaker and recording the response to an acoustic signal. OAEs are less reliable if there is middle ear fluid. Auditory brainstem response (ABR) tests rely on picking up electrical signals on the skin in response to an auditory stimulus. This usually requires general anaesthesia in the newborn, but it may be needed in some circumstances such as

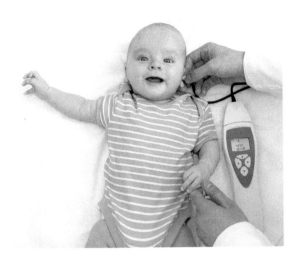

Figure 7.2 Baby undergoing 'screening' by detection of OAEs.

microtia, neonatal meningitis or CMV where the risk of PCHI is high but it may not be picked up by OAEs. Many healthcare systems have an additional 'screening' at the time of school entry, typically around five years of age, using Pure Tone Audiometry or an age-appropriate hearing test. Many children with OME (Chapter 9) are identified in this way.

EARLY INVESTIGATIONS

Investigative protocols differ in different healthcare systems. Once a baby has 'failed' the screening test, early audiological evaluation is essential to confirm or refute (*false positive*) the diagnosis. Once the diagnosis is confirmed, parents will need intensive and ongoing support for what is a devastating and life-changing diagnosis for their newborn baby. Early involvement of an experienced multidisciplinary team makes for the best outcomes.

Initial investigation should focus on determining aetiology, identifying associated conditions, and

planning treatment. Genetic counselling may also be appropriate.

Full audiological and otological assessment and medical evaluation by an experienced paediatric team is essential. Genetic testing, CMV testing, and imaging (CT and/or MRI scanning) are usually arranged. More detailed investigations may be needed depending on the findings, and in consultation with the parents, so that a management plan can be put into effect as soon as possible. The purpose of a screening programme is to ensure early intervention, and the most effective early

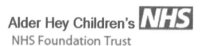

Pure Tone Audiometry Report

Name	
AHnumber	
D.O.B	

Audiometry start time	02/08/2021 16:19:36
Audiometer Serial Number	298362

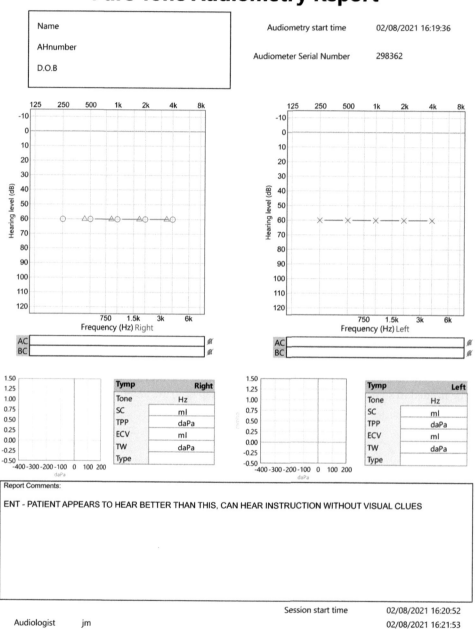

Report Comments:

ENT - PATIENT APPEARS TO HEAR BETTER THAN THIS, CAN HEAR INSTRUCTION WITHOUT VISUAL CLUES

Audiologist   jm

Session start time   02/08/2021 16:20:52
02/08/2021 16:21:53

1

Figure 7.3 Audiogram in a case of functional hearing loss.

intervention is amplification, initially with use of one or more usually two hearing aids. Enormous technological advances in the design and manufacture of hearing aids have taken place in recent decades, and children benefit from hearing aids from as early as the first few weeks of life, i.e. as soon as they can be fitted.

▮ Unilateral hearing loss

Traditional teaching that one ear was entirely sufficient for optimum development of language and communication skills is misplaced. Single-sided deafness (SSD) warrants early identification and active intervention to ensure these children maximise their potential. If recognised, SSD may warrant amplification (usually with conventional hearing aids) and ongoing surveillance, including awareness and support in the home and school environment.

▮ 'Functional' hearing loss

This is probably a better term than 'non-organic hearing loss' as the latter is sometimes used to refer to subjects who feign hearing loss for financial gain (e.g. compensation for alleged noise-induced hearing loss). These children are not 'feigning' deafness and it is counterproductive in the extreme to suggest they are. Adolescents, more often girls, sometimes present with reported hearing loss, often 'confirmed' at pure-tone audiometry (PTA), but with what seems normal responses to conversation and normal speech discrimination in everyday life and without any evidence of ear or other auditory pathology. ABRs are normal (**Figure 7.3**). There may be a background history of psychological distress, anxiety, high academic expectation, school problems or bullying. Treatment is expectant and improvement is usual but the child and family may need psychological referral and support.

▮ Auditory processing disorders

Variously referred to as auditory neuropathy or auditory dysynchrony (AD), the preferred term is *auditory neuropathy spectrum disorders* (ANSDs). This is an 'umbrella' term for a group of conditions characterised by normal OAEs with normal or near normal ABRs. Older children show normal or near-normal PTA but have difficulty processing normal speech. The pathology is uncertain, it is thought to relate to auditory nerve dysfunction but with a normal cochlea. The range of conditions encountered is probably far more complex, in most cases, the aetiology is unknown, and many cases are now acknowledged to have a genetic basis. There is a high incidence of comorbidity, including attention deficit disorder (ADD), ASDs, and apraxia and developmental delay. Amplification may help following rigorous audiological evaluation, but these children require intensive support with early language intervention by skilled teachers to achieve their full potential.

KEY POINTS

- The outcomes for babies with congenital hearing loss have greatly improved, but hearing impairment remains a significant worldwide cause of disability.
- Early recognition and intervention are essential to ensure optimum outcomes for deaf children.
- Children 'at risk' of congenital hearing loss who pass the newborn screening test should be considered for 'surveillance' as they may present with later-onset hearing loss.
- SSD should be recognised so children can be referred early for investigation and rehabilitation.

FURTHER READING

Liming BJ, Carter J, Cheng A et al. International Pediatric Otolaryngology Group (IPOG) consensus recommendations: Hearing loss in the pediatric patient. *Int J Pediatr Otorhinolaryngol.* 2016;90:251–8. doi: 10.1016/j.ijporl.2016.09.016.

NHS. Newborn hearing screening. (Details of the newborn screening programme (UK) and resources for parents.) Available at: https://www.nhs.uk/conditions/baby/newborn-screening/hearing-test/ (accessed 24 January 2022).

Nicolas S, Gallois Y, Calmels MN. Quality of life of children treated for unilateral hearing loss: a systematic review and meta-analysis. *Arch Dis Child.* 2021;106(11):1102–10. doi: 10.1136/archdischild-2020-320389.

Wilson BS, Tucci DL, Merson MH, O'Donoghue GM. Global hearing health care: new findings and perspectives. *The Lancet* 2017;390(10111):2503–15. doi: 10.1016/S0140-6736(17)31073-5.

8 HEARING TESTS

INTRODUCTION

Age-appropriate assessment is essential to the early detection, categorisation and management of hearing impairment in childhood. Degrees of hearing loss are defined in **Table 8.1**. *Objective tests* do not require the cooperation of the child but rely on picking up electrophysiological signals in response to sound. OAE tests – widely used in newborn screening (see Chapter 7) and ABR tests are the main objective tests. ABR involves placing sensors on the child's head to record electrophysiological changes in response to a sound signal fed in via an earphone. The child needs to be asleep and may require sedation or anaesthesia. *Subjective tests* measure a response that the child volunteers when they hear a presented test sound.

Table 8.1 Degrees of hearing loss defined.

Degree of hearing loss	Hearing loss range (dB HL)
Mild	26–40
Moderate	41–55
Moderately severe	56–70
Severe	71–90

BEHAVIOURAL OBSERVATION AUDIOMETRY

Behavioural observation audiometry (BOA) involves recording changes in activity – often head turning – in response to a sound stimulus (*distraction test*). It was widely used in babies up to the age of about 6 months, but objective tests are now generally preferred in this age group.

In a *visual reinforcement audiometry (VRA) test*, sounds of different frequencies and loudness are presented. When the child hears the sound, they turn their head and a 'reward' such as a flashing toy is activated. These tests require a trained and skilled audiometrician and a sound-proofed test room. Incorporating a test into a game that the child learns and enjoys – putting men in a wooden boat in response to a sound stimulus (*play audiometry*) – may be appropriate for toddlers and preschool children who are not old enough for pure-tone audiometry.

Pure-tone audiometry (PTA) is the standard test method for adults and older children. Most children can be taught to undertake PTA from the age of about

DOI: 10.1201/9780429019128-8

4 years onwards, but the test requires concentration and active participation. A series of signals ('pure tones') of different frequencies and at different loudness levels is presented via headphones, and the child indicates when they hear the signal (**Figure 8.1**). A graph is then plotted of loudness against frequency to give an easy-to-read assessment of hearing via air conduction (AC) across a range of frequencies.

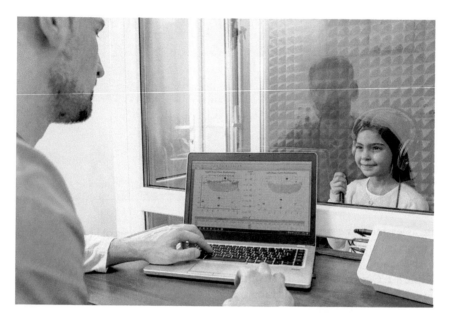

Figure 8.1 Hearing test (PTA) in progress.

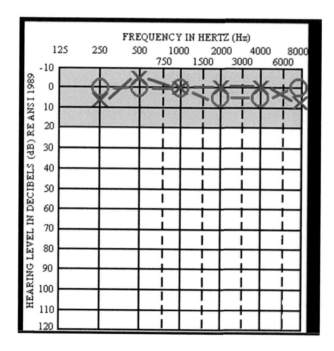

Figure 8.2 Audiogram.

Bone-conduction testing is now performed using a vibrating device (bone conductor) placed on the skin over the mastoid. A significant difference between AC and bone conduction (BC) (air–bone gap) suggests a conductive deafness, as occurs in OME (**Figure 8.2**).

More specialised tests such as *speech discrimination tests* which test the child's capacity to hear words at different loudness levels may be needed in particular situations.

IMPEDANCE AUDIOMETRY (TYMPANOMETRY)

This is not a test of hearing but gives important information about the 'compliance' and by implication the degree of 'stiffness' of the eardrum and middle ear. A small probe in the ear canal emits a tone via a microphone, and a speaker measures the sound reflected from the drum at different levels of air pressure (**Figure 8.3**). In practice, compliance correlates well with the mobility of the eardrum and middle ear. A 'flat' (Type B) tympanogram with reduced middle-ear compliance across a range of air pressures is characteristic of a middle ear effusion. A 'Type C' trace with a negative middle ear pressure peak is highly suggestive of Eustachian tube dysfunction (see Chapter 9).

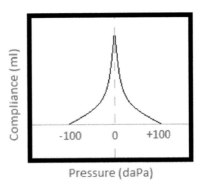

Figure 8.3 Normal tympanogram.

KEY POINTS

- Make sure the chosen test is suitable for the child's developmental age. This is not always the same as the chronological age.
- Tympanometry – with otoscopy and pure tone audiometry – is a helpful adjunct to the diagnosis of OME.

FURTHER READING
NHS guidance for hearing tests for children. Available at: https://www.nhs.uk/conditions/hearing-tests-children/ (accessed 29 March 2022)

9

OTITIS MEDIA WITH EFFUSION

INTRODUCTION

Fluid in the middle ear is an inevitable part of childhood. It occurs during an episode of acute otitis media (AOM) when it causes localised pain and systemic upset, but a painless effusion – usually self-limiting – is a common event in children and, apart from a short period of mild hearing loss, causes no adverse effects.

Otitis media with effusion (OME) is defined as the persistent presence of middle ear fluid for at least 3 months. Most cases resolve with no treatment. The majority of affected children probably do not come to the attention of ORL or audiology professionals.

Persistent OME will need active management and, if untreated, may result in suboptimal educational and cognitive outcomes for the child.

INCIDENCE AND AETIOLOGY

Most children develop OME during the preschool years, with a lower incidence beyond the age of 6 or 7 years. OME may follow an unresolved episode of AOM, but there is not always a history of an earlier acute episode. The effusion is mucinous ('glue ear') or serous and may be sterile. It is thought to be produced by goblet cells in the middle ear and Eustachian tubal mucosa. Eustachian tubal dysfunction has long been implicated as part of the aetiology of OME but, in truth, the cause is not completely understood. There is a seasonal variation, the condition being commoner in the winter months. Exposure to tobacco smoke (passive smoking), respiratory allergy and close contact with other children such as occurs in daycare centres and crèches have been implicated. Breastfeeding seems to offer some protection. Children at particular risk include those with cleft palate, Down syndrome (trisomy 21) and craniofacial disorders. Cystic fibrosis (CF), ciliary dyskinesia and immune dysfunction also predispose to OME. There is increasing interest in the role of 'biofilms' – including in the adenoidal tissue (see Chapter 15) in the pathogenesis of OME.

DOI: 10.1201/9780429019128-9

CLINICAL PRESENTATION AND INVESTIGATIONS

Many children have no symptoms. Some present with hearing loss, noticed at home or at school. Some have earache, a sensation of pressure in the ear or a vague sensation of balance disturbance. Tinnitus is uncommon. Otoscopic appearances can be very variable, but the typical findings are of a bulging translucent drum (**Figure 9.1**), sometimes with bubbles or an air–fluid level. Sometimes – especially in long-standing cases – there may be retraction of the drum onto the ossicles or even the medial wall of the middle ear. The diagnosis is clinical but confirmed by PTA in children who can do a PTA, i.e. usually children over 4 years old, assuming the child has reached the expected developmental milestones and is co-operative. PTA will show a conductive loss (**Figure 9.2**), with an 'air-bone gap' of up to 35 db. A tympanogram will typically show a 'flat' trace (Type B, **Figure 9.3**).

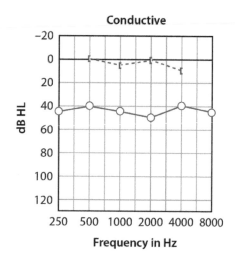

Figure 9.2 PTA showing typical bilateral conductive loss in OME.

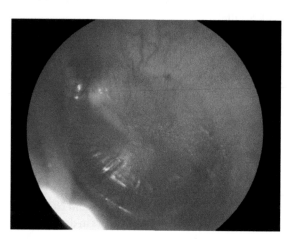

Figure 9.1 Otoscopic view of OME.

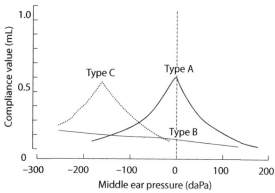

Figure 9.3 Tympanometry is a useful adjunct in the diagnosis of OME. A 'Type b'(flat) trace is typical, but a 'Type c' trace is also commonly found.

MANAGEMENT

Most children with OME will have complete resolution of their effusions without any treatment. All children and their teachers and families will benefit from advice regarding good hearing strategies (**Box 9.1**).

'Watchful' waiting refers to expectant management but with serial observation so that treatment can be offered if the hearing loss is prolonged or becomes especially problematic. Multiple treatment modalities have been subjected to rigorous analysis, but the

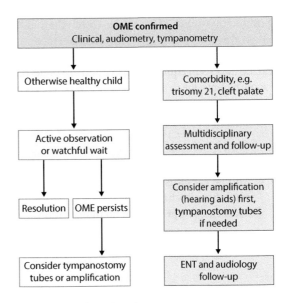

Figure 9.4 Algorithm showing management strategy for OME.

evidence base for treatments other than tympanostomy tubes and amplification (hearing aids) is sparse.

Medical treatments such as antibiotics, mucolytics and antihistamines are largely ineffective. Systemic or intranasal steroids may be of some benefit but have significant side effects. Auto-inflation devices (balloons through which the child can inflate the Eustachian tube using a nozzle introduced to the nose) and the more invasive approach of Eustachian tubal balloon inflation all enjoy some popularity but, in practice, the two most often used modalities of active treatment are *ventilation tubes* and *amplification* (hearing aids). Adjuvant adenoidectomy is recommended in some circumstances, for example, in recurrent cases that need a second insertion of tympanostomy tubes, or if there is an independent reason to recommend adenoidectomy (e.g. recalcitrant allergic rhinitis or persistent rhinosinusitis). Many healthcare systems have well-developed guidelines to help clinicians and parents decide on the best approach, usually suggesting an initial trial of expectant treatment and intervention only if symptoms are persistent (**Figure 9.4**).

The tympanostomy tubes (ventilation tubes or 'vents') most widely used are 'grommets' with 'T-tubes' (**Figure 9.5**) reserved for situations where long-term ventilation of the middle ear is required. Tympanostomy tubes are associated with a risk of permanent perforation of the eardrum, about 2% with grommets but as high as 40% with T-tubes. Troublesome infection and discharge may also complicate the use of ventilation tubes, but these are usually manageable by a short course of ciprofloxacin drops. Tympanosclerosis (scarring with calcified

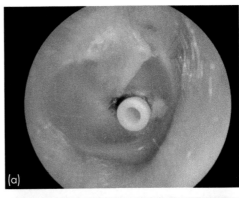

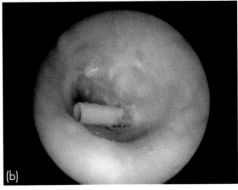

Figure 9.5 Tympanostomy tubes: (a) grommet, (b) T-tube.

deposits in the drum and sometimes within the middle ear) can also occur as a reaction to ventilation tubes.

Hearing aids seem equally effective and are preferred by some parents due to the long-term adverse effects of tympanostomy tubes, but many children are reluctant to use hearing aids. They are usually recommended where OME is expected to run a prolonged course such as in children with Down syndrome and in OME associated with cleft-palate.

KEY POINTS

- Middle ear effusion is almost universal at some time in children.
- Most cases improve with no intervention.

FURTHER READING

NICE. Otitis media with effusion: What information and advice can I give to parents of children with otitis media with effusion (OME)? Available at: https://cks.nice.org.uk/topics/otitis-media-with-effusion/management/management/#advice-to-parents (accessed 20 January 2022).

10 ACUTE OTITIS MEDIA

INTRODUCTION

Acute inflammatory changes in the middle ear are an almost universal feature of childhood and most children will have had one or more episodes of acute otitis media (AOM) by their second birthday. Infection is typically short-lived and self-limiting, but AOM can have serious sequelae and complications.

PATHOGENESIS

Infection is usually initially viral. The middle ear is part of the upper respiratory tract and is in communication with the pharynx via the Eustachian tube, hence the common viral pathogens – parainfluenza virus, *respiratory syncytial virus* (RSV), coronaviruses, etc. – may all be implicated. The mucosa of the middle ear and Eustachian tube become suffused and oedematous, with hyperaemia of the tympanic membrane, and an increase in secretions into the middle ear, which may become tense and engorged causing the child pain and distress. Often, this resolves quickly but bacterial superinfection can supervene due to the proliferation of pyogenic organisms such as *Streptococcus pyogenes*, *Staphylococcus aureus* and *Moraxella catharhalis*. This causes increased pain, tense swelling, with an inflammatory exudate into the middle ear and the mastoid air cells. The tympanic membrane may perforate, usually accompanied by a purulent external discharge and some relief of pain. The possible outcomes of AOM are shown in **Figure 10.1**.

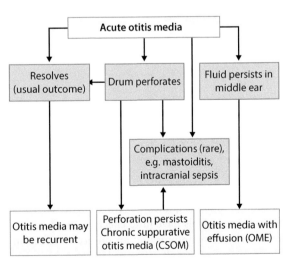

Figure 10.1 Algorithm showing outcomes of AOM.

DOI: 10.1201/9780429019128-10

PREDISPOSING FACTORS

Most children who develop AOM are otherwise healthy, and ear infections are an expected part of childhood. Children at greater risk include those with immune dysfunction such as children receiving chemotherapy, children with specific disorders of immunity and children with CF. AOM is to a degree seasonal and is more prevalent in the autumn and winter months. Breastfeeding offers some protection, and children looked after in day-care centres seem to be more at risk, presumably due to earlier exposure to environmental pathogens in the community. Passive exposure to tobacco smoke is a risk factor, as are a number of medical conditions (e.g. cleft palate). The role of the adenoids is disputed, but it seems likely that adenoids may harbour and shed bacteria that colonise and proliferate in the Eustachian tube, hence the place of adenoidectomy in the management of recalcitrant cases of recurrent acute otitis media (RAOM).

DIAGNOSIS AND INVESTIGATIONS

AOM implies the presence of pathogens in the middle ear but, in practice, the diagnosis is almost always made clinically with no attempt to identify or culture the offending organisms. Otalgia, pyrexia and a distressed child with otoscopic features of inflammation (reddened bulging drum, **Figure 10.2**) are the usual findings. Other conditions such as tonsillitis, 'teething' or uncomplicated respiratory infection can have similar features, and this diagnostic uncertainty has made evaluation of the evidence for treatment, particularly antimicrobial therapy, very difficult.

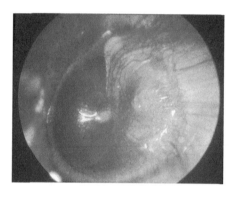

Figure 10.2 Otoscopic view in AOM.

MANAGEMENT

AOM is painful, and the first requirement is to make sure the child has adequate analgesia. Paracetamol, stepping up to ibuprofen if needed, with good hydration and general support will usually be adequate. The role of antimicrobial therapy is still not fully established or agreed upon despite numerous studies and the publication of multiple guidelines. The evidence suggests that antimicrobials have little effect on the duration or severity of symptoms and an uncertain effect on the frequency of complications or long-term sequelae. Despite increasing concern regarding the overenthusiastic use of antibiotics and the development of resistance to standard antibiotics in the community, many clinicians, and parents, are understandably uneasy about withholding antibiotics, especially if there is evidence of bacterial infection (e.g. severe pain or purulent discharge). Impending or actual complications are, of course, an absolute indication for antibiotics, and the first choice based on known pathogens is usually amoxycillin, with a cephalosporin as second line.

Surgery has a limited role, but myringotomy to release a tense bulging eardrum may be considered in recalcitrant cases where there has been little or no response to medical therapy, or where complications have developed.

This is not well defined, but most authorities would accept that more than three documented episodes of AOM in a 6-month period warrant the term 'RAOM'. Expectant treatment is best, if at all possible, but this condition can cause a great deal of distress to parents and children, and there is some evidence to support the use of long-term prophylactic antibiotics. Tympanostomy tubes (grommets) are sometimes considered, but the evidence is unclear and there is no doubt that grommets are associated with specific risks including recurrent mucopurulent discharge and long-term tympanic membrane perforation. Adenoidectomy may help remove the aggregated communities of bacteria or 'biofilms' thought to be responsible for recurrent infections.

FURTHER READING

Suzuki HG, Dewez JE, Nijman RG, Yeung S. Clinical practice guidelines for acute otitis media in children: a systematic review and appraisal of European national guidelines. *BMJ Open*. 2020;10(5):e035343. doi: 10.1136/bmjopen-2019-035343.

KEY POINTS

- There is very little evidence to support the routine use of antibiotics in uncomplicated otitis media in children. Antibiotics make little difference to symptoms or complications. A 'delayed' or 'back-up' prescription may be appropriate.
- Although rare, complications of otitis media can be devastating. Advise parents to seek medical advice if symptoms persist or deteriorate, or if the child becomes systemically unwell.

11 CHRONIC OTITIS MEDIA

INTRODUCTION

Chronic otitis media (COM) refers to a spectrum of conditions including chronic suppurative otitis media (CSOM) in which the eardrum is perforated with (*active*) or without (*quiescent* or *inactive*) ear discharge, localised retraction pockets of the eardrum, and the more destructive condition *cholesteatoma*. COM may follow one or more episodes of acute otitis media (AOM) but may also arise without a definite antecedent history of acute infection.

PREVALENCE

COM, particularly perforation of the eardrum, is a common finding in children, but the majority of perforations occur in the course of an acute infection and heal well. Ethnicity is an important factor, with COM occurring much more frequently in indigenous Australians, native Americans and children of Inuit heritage. Socioeconomic factors, poverty, deprivation and poor primary healthcare can contribute, and prevalence is much higher in the developing world where CSOM is an important public health problem and a significant cause of childhood deafness. Perforations are found in up to 2% of children who have had tympanostomy tubes (grommets).

CLINICAL FEATURES

Discharge, usually mucopurulent, and deafness are the main presenting symptoms. COM may be 'silent' and only detected on otoscopic examination. Pyogenic organisms (*Streptococcus pyogenese*, *Staphylococcus aureus* and *Moraxella catharalis*) can cause a profuse mucopurulent discharge, but anaerobic organisms such as are more often found in cholesteatoma (*Pseudomonas aeruginosa*) may cause a scanty and sometimes fetid discharge. Occasionally, COM can present with complications such as facial palsy and intracranial sepsis.

DOI: 10.1201/9780429019128-11

THE PERFORATED EARDRUM

Perforation of the eardrum may follow a single epi-sode of AOM, or there may be a history of recur-rent AOM. Some cases are iatrogenic, usually as a complication of tympanostomy tubes, and about 2% of cases of tympanostomy tubes are complicated by long-term perforation.

The site of the perforation is important, as a central perforation (**Figure 11.1**) is less likely to be associ-ated with cholesteatoma than a perforation in the attic region, with associated bone destruction, but the older classification of perforations as 'attico-antral' or 'tubo-tympanic' is too simplistic and no longer considered useful. A dry inactive or quiescent perforation is often asymptomatic and may only be suspected or discovered at otoscopic examination. Many perforations heal, usually with no adverse effects but sometimes leaving residual scarring or retraction of the tympanic membrane, often with calcification – 'tympanosclerosis' – of the drum or the middle ear structures (**Figure 11.2**). What is really important in planning management is whether there is a cholesteatoma, hence the division of CSOM into CSOM *without* cholesteatoma (**Figure 11.1**) and CSOM *with* cholesteatoma (**Figure 11.3**).

A perforation may be active or inactive. A 'wet' perforation will discharge, usually mucopurulent

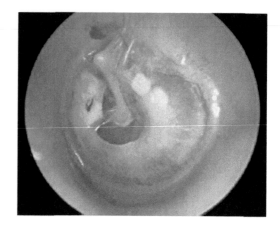

Figure 11.2 Old healed perforation. A thin mem-brane has closed the perforation but there is cal-cification of the surrounding parts of the eardrum (tympanosclerosis).

material, sometimes more or less constantly but more often with long spells where there is no dis-charge. Hearing loss is variable and, if there is no ossicular disease, it may be very minimal.

A 'wet' perforation with intermittent or constant discharge should be managed initially with intensive medical treatment. Regular aural toilet in the form of cleaning of debris, gentle suction and the use of

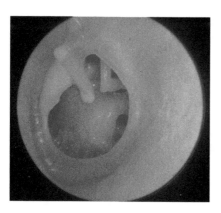

Figure 11.1 Dry central perforation. Inactive or qui-escent CSOM.

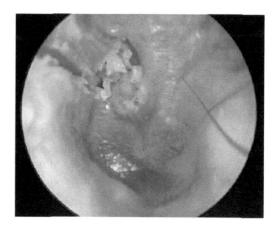

Figure 11.3 Attic perforation with underlying cholesteatoma.

antibiotic drops (ciprofloxacin) with strict adherence to keeping the ear dry and free of external contaminants is often enough to dry up the infection.

A dry inactive perforation may need no intervention. If the child is symptomatic (i.e. with a significant hearing loss or recurrent troublesome discharge), surgery in the form of tympanoplasty (myringoplasty) to close the perforation, usually with native fascia, may be considered. Children who are especially keen on watersports also warrant consideration of surgery. Several techniques are described, the most popular relying on temporalis fascia harvested from behind the ear and used as an 'underlay' to form a scaffold over which new epithelium grows to close the defect. The optimum age for tympanoplasty is debated, but most otologists wait until the child is about 7–8 years old, by which time Eustachian tubal function will have improved making for better long-term outcomes.

RETRACTION POCKETS

Retraction of all or part of the eardrum is a common sequel of Eustachian tubal dysfunction and may complicate both AOM and OME. Small retraction pockets cause little in the way of adverse effects, particularly if the middle ear is well ventilated, but more severe retraction can obliterate the middle ear space and cause significant conductive deafness, with the potential for ingress of squamous epithelium into the middle ear cleft with erosion of bone and formation of cholesteatoma. Otologists differ in their approach to management of retractions, with some preferring a 'wait and see' approach except for the most extreme cases, and some preferring early intervention. Surgical excision, with or without cartilaginous reinforcement of the resulting defect (tympanoplasty), ventilation of the middle ear (tympanostomy tubes) and attention to Eustachian tubal dysfunction (adenoidectomy, balloon dilatation) are all advocated. The evidence base for any treatment approach is uncertain.

CHOLESTEATOMA

Keratinising squamous epithelium is not normally present in the middle ear and, if a mass of such tissue is found in the middle ear and/or the mastoid air cells, it is termed a *cholesteatoma*. It is liable to recurrent infection and is potentially erosive, involving the ossicles and surrounding structures including the tegmen, facial nerve and petrous apex. The precise aetiology is unknown but the more common acquired form is thought to occur as a consequence of persistent ingrowth of epithelium from the external ear beyond the annulus and into the middle ear cleft. It may begin as a retraction pocket and is associated with Eustachian tubal dysfunction.

Most cholesteatomas are acquired, but congenital cholesteatoma is well recognised in children and presents as a mass behind an intact eardrum. It may be due to ectopic cell rests and can involve the petrous apex with or without middle ear involvement.

Cholesteatoma is similar histologically in adults and children, but there are important differences in pathogenesis and behaviour. Most otologists will describe paediatric cholesteatoma as being more aggressive and more destructive, such that early intervention and prolonged follow-up are essential. The child's Eustachian tubal function may be worse, making treatment more difficult, and the greater pneumatisation of the mastoid air cells in children makes for more extensive spread and more challenging surgery.

Diagnosis is clinical, but imaging (CT scanning) is highly recommended to assess the extent, look for bony destruction and plan surgery (**Figure 11.4**).

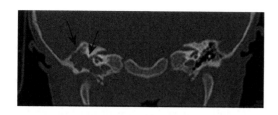

Figure 11.4 CT scan showing extensive cholesteatoma with bone erosion (arrows).

Treatment of cholesteatoma is surgical, and the special challenges in children are such that experienced surgeons with access to good imaging, oto-endoscopic techniques as needed and intraoperative facial nerve monitoring should undertake this surgery. Various techniques are described, with some otologists preferring to keep the canal wall intact (canal wall up, CWU), and some preferring the better intra-operative access of the canal wall down (CWD) approach. These techniques are described and evaluated in more detail in standard otology textbooks.

FURTHER READING

Schilder AGM, Marom T, Bhutta MF et al. Panel 7: Otitis media: treatment and complications. *Otolaryngol Head Neck Surg.* 2017;156(4_suppl):S88–S105. doi: 10.1177/0194599816633697. PMID: 28372534

12 SURGERY FOR CHILDHOOD HEARING LOSS

INTRODUCTION

The role of the surgeon in managing children with permanent childhood hearing impairment is now largely focused on *implantation otology*, i.e. the use of implants to the skull or the ear to channel acoustic signals to the auditory nerve and auditory cortex. There have been enormous strides in this area in recent years with continuing improvements in technology and outcomes. Only the essential principles of the main varieties of implants are presented here.

Where children need amplification (e.g. in bilateral conductive, sensorineural and mixed loss and in many cases of unilateral loss), the first option will be to use a hearing aid. A bone-conducting hearing device (BCHD) – usually a bone-anchored hearing aid (BAHA) – is considered where there is microtia, chronic otitis externa or in SSD where the rationale is to divert sound to the contralateral ear via the skull bones. In general, BCHDs depend on good cochlear function, and many patients who have used both traditional hearing aids and BCHDs will express a preference for BCHDs. For children where a BAHA is planned, the skull bone needs to have developed so that it is thick enough to accommodate the implant, usually at about 2 years of age. A Softband® can be a useful way of ensuring good amplification until the child is a little older.

BONE-CONDUCTING HEARING DEVICES

BCHDs may be *implantable* – i.e. requiring surgery to position all or part of the device – or *non-implantable*.

■ Non-implantable BCHDs

All these work on the principle of sound conduction transmitted transcutaneously through the skull bones to the cochlea using a device worn on the head. They are usually well tolerated in babies and younger children but some children can be very sensitive to objects over or around the head. Non-implantable BCHDs are useful in microtia, chronic otitis externa and sometimes in single-sided sensorineural deafness. A trial of a non-implantable BCHD is nearly always

DOI: 10.1201/9780429019128-12

recommended before progressing to an implantable BCHD.

Examples of non-implantable BCHDs include:

- Softband® (**Figure 12.1**).
- MED-EL ADHEAR® *Adhesive* – an adhesive adapter attached to the skin behind the ear and a sound processor. The sound processor 'clicks' on to the adapter. Children who don't tolerate a headband may find this easier to wear (**Figure 12.2**).
- BCHD attached to spectacle frames.

▌ Implantable BCHDs

These are of two main types, percutaneous and transcutaneous.

Percutaneous devices involve an osseo-integrated implant which projects through the skin so as to anchor an 'abutment' to which a processor – which amplifies and conducts sound – is attached. Acoustic energy is transmitted to the skull bones and thence to the middle ear and cochlea. A BAHA (**Figure 12.3**) is one such device. It is 'passive' in that the processor simply amplifies and transmits the sound energy.

In the alternative *transcutaneous devices*, the processor is not directly attached to bone but attaches to a magnet under the skin. The MED-EL® Bonebridge system is one such device. The parts embedded under the skin bring about vibration of the skull bone via the implanted 'transducer'. The external 'processor' – attached to the skin via a magnet – picks up the sound, converts it to electrical signals and transmits them to the implanted parts ('transducer') and thence to the skull bones and the cochlea where they are received as sound. This is an 'active' rather than a passive device and an 'under-the-skin' system with no open scars or wounds (**Figure 12.4**).

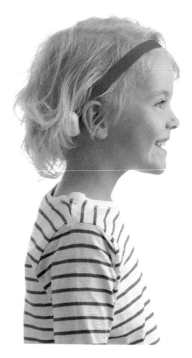

Figure 12.1 Child using a Softband®

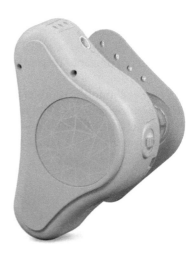

Figure 12.2 MED-EL ADHEAR®, a transcutaneous BCHD.

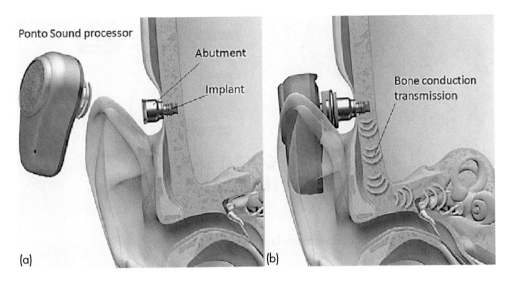

Figure 12.3 (a,b) A BAHA and how it effects transmission.

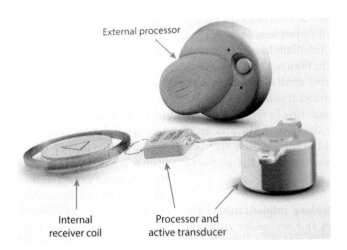

Figure 12.4 MED-EL® Bonebridge. The external processor connects with the internal components transcutaneously via a magnet. The internal processor and transducer are completely covered (i.e. with no parts projecting through the skin).

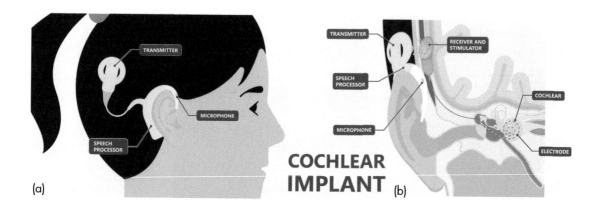

Figure 12.5 (a,b) Components of a cochlear implant.

COCHLEAR IMPLANTATION

Cochlear implantation has revolutionised the treatment of severe and profound hearing loss in children. The cochlear implant (CI) is an implantable device that electrically stimulates the cochlear spiral ganglion cells when the hair cells are not functioning effectively, such that neural impulses are transmitted along the auditory nerve to the cortex where they are processed to produce awareness of sound including speech intelligibility. The components of a CI are shown in **Figure 12.5**. There is an external device (processor) consisting of a microphone, speech processor and transmitter coil. The internal component is made up of a receiver/stimulator which picks up the signal from the processor and generates electrical impulses which are then delivered via an electrode array to the auditory nerve.

The indications for cochlear implantation have widened in recent years and are under constant review, but any child with confirmed severe or profound hearing impairment may be eligible. Conventional hearing aids are tried in the first instance, and the child is referred to a multidisciplinary team for full audiometric, medical and radiological assessment. Early implantation (as early as the first year of life) is crucial to the development of good speech discrimination. This is because of the phenomenon of 'neural plasticity' within the central nervous system, with a far greater capacity for adaptability in the immature auditory neural networks including the brainstem. There is increasing evidence now to support the practice of bilateral implantation and to consider implantation for SSD as devices become more sophisticated.

Surgical techniques have improved in recent years with implantation taking place largely in designated centres where there is an experienced multidisciplinary team. Intensive support in the postoperative period under the supervision of a skilled audiology team is essential to a successful outcome. Complications are uncommon and include very rare instances of facial nerve trauma, but more commonly issues with skin flaps which may mean the device has to be removed or re-implanted. Long-term device failure is uncommon but regular follow-up and surveillance of children is needed post implantation. Intensive supportive rehabilitation under the supervision of a dedicated team including audiologists and teachers is vital to long-term success, especially in the early days following surgery.

AUDITORY BRAINSTEM IMPLANT

An auditory brainstem implant (ABI) is a device which is implanted in the cochlear nucleus in the brainstem rather than the inner ear. It may be useful in very a small number of circumstances when a CI is unsuitable, such as in cases of neurofibromatosis type 2 (NF2), where the cochlear nerves have been irreparably damaged. Experience with ABIs in children is very limited.

MIDDLE EAR IMPLANTS

The idea of a device within the middle ear to augment hearing is an attractive alternative to conventional hearing aids, and a few such devices are now available. 'Active' surgically implanted middle ear implants (MEIs) may stimulate the ossicles or the inner ear. Experience in children is very limited, but MEIs may become more useful as technology improves.

KEY POINTS

- Surgery for PCHI is now largely focused on implantation.
- Technological developments in this field are rapidly advancing, and new techniques and devices regularly become available.
- Cochlear implantation has transformed outcomes for children with congenital hearing loss.

FURTHER READING

Bagatto M, Gordey D, Brewster L et al. Clinical consensus document for fitting non-surgical transcutaneous bone conduction hearing devices to children. *Int J Audiol.* 2021;1–8. doi: 10.1080/14992027.2021.1939449.

Gordey D, Bagatto M. Fitting bone conduction hearing devices to children: audiological practices and challenges. *Int J Audiol.* 2021;60(5):385–92. doi: 10.1080/14992027.2020.1814970.

NICE. Guidance: Cochlear implants for children and adults with severe to profound deafness. Available at: https://www.nice.org.uk/guidance/ta566 (accessed 24 January 2022).

Simon F, Roman S, Truy E et al. Guidelines (short version) of the French Society of Otorhinolaryngology (SFORL) on pediatric cochlear implant indications. *Eur Ann Otorhinolaryngol Head Neck Dis.* 2019;136(5):385–91. doi: 10.1016/j.anorl.2019.05.018.

13 BALANCE DISORDERS

INTRODUCTION

Children and adolescents frequently complain of 'dizziness', or cause concern to their parents because they are clumsy, fall easily or seem to struggle with their balance. The great majority of causes are benign, but clinicians need to be aware of 'red flag' symptoms and signs that warrant urgent further investigation. Reasons for 'dysequilibrium' are legion and, while clinicians need to be vigilant, serious progressive pathology in children does not often present in this way. Some 'red flag' presentations are shown in **Box 13.1**.

Many cases are due to normal maturation of the physiological systems that contribute to maintaining balance; the vestibular apparatus does not fully mature until well into the teenage years. Migrainous disorders are far more common in children than was previously acknowledged and often present atypically, not always with a headache. True vestibular disorders in children are uncommon and, when they occur, they tend to be self-limiting and characterised by early and effective compensation. Most presentations of 'dizziness' are due to non-vestibular pathology. Some causes of balance dysfunction in children are shown in **Box 13.2**.

Box 13.1 'Red flags' in children with 'dizziness'

- Persistent or recurrent headache
- Persistent or recurrent vomiting
- Suspected seizures
- Focal neurological symptoms/signs e.g. 'tingling', numbness
  - Abnormal eye movements
  - Blurred vision
  - Change in behaviour
- Cardiac symptoms e.g. syncope, palpitations

Box 13.2 Some common causes of imbalance

With hearing loss

- OME
- CSOM
- Surgery to brain or ear
- Ototoxic drugs

Without hearing loss

- Migraine (includes benign paroxysmal vertigo of childhood, BPVC)
- Vestibular neuronitis
- Functional disorders

DOI: 10.1201/9780429019128-13

CLINICAL PRESENTATION

Take a detailed and thorough history. The duration of symptoms can be of great diagnostic help. 'Dizziness' lasting for a few seconds suggests benign paroxysmal positional vertigo (BPPV) but this is rare in children. Episodes lasting a few hours may be due to migraine, or benign paroxysmal vertigo of childhood (BPVC) which is now thought to be a variant of migraine. *Vestibular neuronitis* and *acute labyrinthitis* symptoms last for a few days, but compensation in children is much more rapid than in adults. Associated symptoms can help narrow the diagnosis; nausea and vomiting suggest vestibular pathology but may occur in migraine. Neurological features such as seizures or cranial nerve palsies are alarming and warrant urgent investigation to rule out intracranial pathology. Anxiety, depression and eating disorders may be associated with balance dysfunction. 'Functional' (or 'psychogenic' vertigo as it used to be known) is common, and the rapid hormonal changes of adolescence can often be accompanied by symptoms of 'dizziness' caused by postural (orthostatic) hypotension. Adolescence is also a time when young people may be subject to exam pressures, bullying, intense social media activity and sometimes family disharmony, all of which can manifest as somatic symptoms including balance disorders.

Hearing loss is a feature of otitis media, and hearing loss with tinnitus occurs in Menière's disease, but this is rare in children. OME is frequently associated with clumsiness, falls, and 'dizziness'.

EXAMINATION AND INVESTIGATION

Clinical examination starts as the child enters the consulting room. Observe their gait, posture and motor function. A thorough ENT examination is important, particularly otoscopy, and a basic neurological examination to include evaluation of the function of the cranial nerves is helpful. Look for nystagmus. Any findings that suggest a focal neurological lesion warrant urgent investigation and referral, including imaging (CT/MRI scanning) of the head. Age-appropriate audiometry and tympanometry are an integral part of a routine ENT examination. More sophisticated investigations are not always needed unless dictated by the findings of initial clinical assessment. Specialist clinics offer vestibular function tests.

MANAGEMENT

Once sinister or progressive causes have been excluded, parents and children are usually happy to be reassured that there is no ominous pathology. Most conditions are managed expectantly and will resolve. Advice and counselling with regard to migraine, with an emphasis on reassurance and avoiding 'triggers', may be all that is needed. Avoid medication if you can, but drugs such as pizotifen and propranolol have a place in controlling severe symptoms. Very troublesome migraine may require prophylaxis and medication to subdue the acute attacks, especially if there is accompanying headache.

Specialist vestibular clinics will offer specific strategies such as the Epley maneouvre for BPPV and vestibular rehabilitation exercises for prolonged vestibular failure. If imbalance is secondary to otitis media, the treatment is that of the primary condition (e.g. grommets for OME and tympanomastoid surgery for cholesteatoma).

KEY POINTS

- Parents and clinicians worry that symptoms of 'dysequilibrium' can be due to serious intracranial pathology, but this is extremely uncommon. Brain tumours very rarely present with imbalance as the sole symptom.
- Apart from audiometry, few if any investigations are needed to evaluate the 'dizzy' child.
- Imaging is rarely helpful unless there is a definite and specific indication.
- Vestibular migraine (or a migraine variant) is the commonest cause of episodes of imbalance in children.
- Avoid medication if at all possible. Most cases are self-limiting.
- The main role of the clinician is to take a careful history, exclude sinister pathology and provide reassurance and support.
- OME is frequently accompanied by balance dysfunction. The mechanism is unknown.

FURTHER READING

van de Berg R, Widdershoven J, Bisdorff A et al. Vestibular migraine of childhood and recurrent vertigo of childhood: diagnostic criteria consensus document of the Committee for the Classification of Vestibular Disorders of the Bárány Society and the International Headache Society. *J Vestib Res.* 2021;31(1):1–9. doi: 10.3233/VES-200003.

Ratnayake S, Crunkhorn R, Wong J, Dasgupta S. Vestibular migraine in children. *Audacity Magazine.* 2021;March Edition:30-33. Available at: https://cloud.3dissue.net/30176/30074/30346/49789/# (accessed 6 June 2022)

www.jvr-web.org/images/ICVD-Recurrent-Vertigo-of-Childhood-Diagnostic-Criteria-V20.pdf

14 FACIAL PALSY

INTRODUCTION

The facial nerve is far more superficial in children than in adults. This makes it more vulnerable to trauma including operative injuries. As the mastoid process is rudimentary in the newborn and in early childhood, the intratemporal portion of the nerve is much more exposed than in adults and is especially at risk from a low post-aural incision (**Figure 14.1**). Children with Down syndrome or craniofacial deformity may have particularly complex or unusual facial nerve anatomy, making tympanomastoid surgery in this group especially challenging.

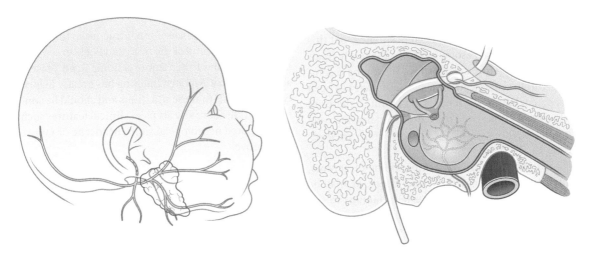

Figure 14.1 Anatomy of the facial nerve in an infant. (a) Intra-temporal course. The mastoid process is higher and less well developed than in the adult. (b) Extra-temporal course. The posterior auricular nerve and the nerve to the digastric branch off, and within the substance of the parotid gland, the nerve divides into the motor branches to the muscles of facial expression. The nerve here is more superficial than in the adult, and vulnerable to injury.

DOI: 10.1201/9780429019128-14

AETIOLOGY

Facial palsy is much less common in children than in adults. Both congenital and acquired aetiologies are described (**Box 14.1**).

Box 14.1 Common aetiologies

- Idiopathic (Bell's palsy)
- Trauma (includes iatrogenic, birth trauma)
- Otitis media
- Congenital
- Intracranial mass

▊ Acquired palsy

As in adults, the commonest cause is *Bell's palsy*, or idiopathic facial paralysis. This usually comes on over a few days but may only be noticed as a 'sudden' presentation, progressing to a complete palsy which then recovers, typically over a period of days or weeks. It is almost always unilateral. A viral aetiology with inflammatory swelling of the perineural tissues in the region of the stylomastoid foramen leading to neuropraxia has been postulated, but this is unproven. There is some evidence that early treatment with systemic corticosteroids hastens resolution. Antiviral medication such as acyclovir has been advocated, but the evidence is uncertain. If there are no unusual clinical features and the palsy recovers completely, investigations are not generally needed.

Trauma may be caused by temporal bone fractures, usually as part of a serious head injury, or may be iatrogenic, for instance inadvertent damage to the nerve during tympanomastoid surgery, parotidectomy or surgery to the neck including excision of lymph nodes or a pharyngeal arch anomaly. Facial palsy is a devastating complication with profound and life-long implications for the child and family and it is not an acceptable outcome for any but the most serious indications for surgery (e.g. malignant disease).

If the nerve is traumatised during surgery, it may simply be 'bruised' (neuropraxia), in which case it will recover. Remove any source of pressure on the nerve including packing/dressings in the ear and protect the eye while awaiting recovery. If the nerve is severed, the outcome is poor even with repair.

A *facial palsy evident in the newborn* may be due to birth trauma. This can complicate a difficult forceps delivery, or in some instances a traumatic non-instrumental vaginal delivery where there is excessive pressure from the mother's sacral promontory on the baby's skull. Unravelling the precise cause can be difficult and may lead to medicolegal disputes; a congenital facial palsy of unknown aetiology presents in a similar way but rarely recovers.

Otitis media can be complicated by facial palsy. AOM with an intact drum can cause a neuropraxia, especially if the bony covering of the nerve is incomplete (dehiscent). Although alarming, and a cause of great distress to parents, facial palsy complicating an AOM almost always recovers. A facial palsy in CSOM is more ominous and suggests erosion of the bony canal covering the nerve. This is an indication for early surgery.

Rarely, *malignant disease* – an intracranial tumour, a rhabdomyosarcoma of the head and neck, or leukaemic infiltration of the temporal bone – can present as a facial palsy. Modern imaging has greatly helped early diagnosis in these situations and should be considered if there are any atypical clinical features such as associated neurological signs, headache or failure to improve.

▊ Congenital facial palsy

'Obstetric' palsy has been alluded to above.

Isolated or multiple cranial nerve palsies including facial palsy occur for no apparent reason, and facial palsy is an important component of some childhood syndromes including Moebius syndrome, Poland syndrome and some cases of CHARGE syndrome (see Chapter 3).

Hemifacial microsomia (as in Goldenhar's syndrome) describes a spectrum of anomalies affecting one side of the face causing both functional and aesthetic asymmetry.

Neonatal asymmetric crying facies presents as asymmetry of the lower lip when the baby cries. It may be a manifestation of facial nerve dysfunction and occurs in 0.6% of live births.

MANAGEMENT OF FACIAL PALSY

Take a careful history, including a birth history, and examine the child with an emphasis on looking for neurological findings, particularly in the other cranial nerves. Otoscopy and, where possible, audiological evaluation are important. Document the severity of the paresis and record the pattern of movement of each of the regions of the face (i.e. the upper, middle and lower parts).

Look carefully at the eye in case there is evidence of early corneal damage or conjunctivitis. If there are unusual clinical features or any suggestion of a mass, imaging can be immensely helpful. MRI with gadolinium enhancement is ideal, if available, and will show the architecture of the nerve from the brainstem to the intraparotid branches.

Early treatment should focus on protecting the eye. Children may not tolerate an eyepatch, but a little tape over the eyelids at night can help to reduce the risk of exposure of the cornea. If you make the diagnosis of Bell's palsy early, then oral steroids for a few days may be worthwhile, as may the addition of acyclovir.

Long-term management of established facial palsy is complex. Muscle and fascial slings and a variety of nerve and muscle reanimation techniques including nerve transfers/anastomoses, nerve repairs and free grafts are used, usually in specialised multidisciplinary team clinics.

KEY POINTS

- Facial palsy due to AOM almost always recovers completely.
- Make sure to protect the cornea, especially at night.

FURTHER READING

Psillas G, Antoniades E, Ieridou F, Constantinidis J. Facial nerve palsy in children: a retrospective study of 124 cases. *J Paediatr Child Health.* 2019;55(3):299–304. doi: 10.1111/jpc.14190.

15

THE PHARYNX AND ORAL CAVITY

INTRODUCTION

The lymphoid tissue of the pharynx surrounds the entrance to the aerodigestive tract. The palatine tonsils, the adenoids and the lingual tonsils collectively constitute *Waldeyer's ring*. The lymphoid follicles that make up these structures are composed of B and T cells and their function is to help develop both cell-mediated and humoral immunity. They are prone to recurrent infection in childhood; tonsillectomy and adenoidectomy remain among the commonest surgical procedures performed in children.

ACUTE PHARYNGITIS AND TONSILLITIS

Viral infection of the pharynx with acute enlargement of the tonsils is an almost universal part of childhood. Pain, difficulty swallowing, fever and enlarged tender neck nodes with erythema and swelling of the tonsils are the presenting features. Acute viral infections are usually self-limiting. Any of the common upper respiratory viruses (rhinoviruses, adenoviruses, coronaviruses) can be responsible, with the *Epstein Barr virus* (EBV) causing a particularly severe form of acute pharyngitis especially in adolescents (*infectious mononucleosis*). Bacterial infection is generally with one of the common pyogenic organisms, including group A beta-haemolytic *Streptococcus pyogenes* (GABHS), *Haemophilus influenzae*, *Streptococcus pneumomiae*. Symptoms are more severe, with marked pain, malaise and sometimes an exudate on the tonsils (**Figure 15.1**). Anaerobic organisms can be implicated in severe infections, particularly if quinsy (peritonsillar abscess) develops.

Diagnosis of acute tonsillitis is largely clinical, and most children are managed in primary care settings rather than by ORL specialists. Acute tonsillitis can usually be managed with symptomatic treatment,

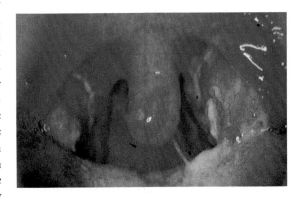

Figure 15.1 Acute tonsillitis.

DOI: 10.1201/9780429019128-15

i.e. analgesics (paracetamol), fluids and observation for signs of deterioration. Resolution is the norm with or without antibiotic treatment but, if antibiotics are deemed appropriate, penicillin is effective against most of the common causative organisms.

Some cases of tonsillitis progress to complications. These include spread of infection to the tissue planes beyond the pharynx (quinsy, parapharyngeal abscess, retropharyngeal abscess), severe airway obstruction and, rarely, generalised septicaemia (see Chapter 5).

NON-INFLAMMATORY CONDITIONS OF THE TONSILS

As the tonsils are composed of lymphoid tissue, they may be the site of presentation of a lymphoma, or a non-lymphoid malignancy in the head and neck. Asymmetry in the size of the tonsils is common in younger children, especially following one or more episodes of tonsillitis, and can cause concern and alarm to both doctors and parents. In the great majority of cases this is harmless but, if there is suspicion of a lymphoma, then tonsillectomy for histology is warranted.

The tonsils are often invaginated by multiple deep crypts, in which cheesy debris and sometimes food particles or even calcified material (tonsilloliths) can collect. Tonsillar debris may contribute to halitosis. Teenagers in particular can find this so distressing that it warrants consideration of a tonsillectomy, even if there is no history of recurrent sore throats.

Gross enlargement of the tonsils can compromise swallowing and contribute to obstructive sleep apnoea (OSA) (see Chapter 16).

Occasionally, the tonsil can be the source of recurrent spontaneous bleeds due to prominent fragile vessels on the mucosal surface. This can be so severe as to warrant tonsillectomy.

Immune complex disorders in childhood (e.g. post-streptococcal glomerulonephritis and rheumatic fever) due to tonsillitis were important causes of renal failure and mitral and aortic valvular heart disease in the past but are far less often seen in modern practice.

TONSILLECTOMY

The indications for tonsillectomy have become more sharply defined in recent years. Many healthcare systems and national ORL societies have guidelines to help parents and clinicians make good evidence-based decisions. Recurrent tonsillitis remains the commonest reason for tonsillectomy in childhood. Most clinicians would offer tonsillectomy to children who fulfil the criteria in accordance with the Scottish Intercollegiate Guidelines Network (SIGN) guidelines (**Box 15.1**). One of the difficulties is that ORL doctors are presented with a child who has a history of episodes of sore throat that have been managed by the primary care team, and it is not always certain that the child has had true tonsillitis.

> **Box 15.1 SIGN guidelines for tonsillectomy (recurrent tonsillitis)**
> - Episodes due to tonsillitis
> - Episodes disabling and prevent normal functioning
> - Seven episodes in preceding year *or*
> - Five episodes in each of preceding 2 years *or*
> - Three episodes in each of preceding 3 years

Mild viral pharyngitis, even if recurrent, is not a good indication for surgery, hence the importance of a careful history to enquire about neck nodes, fever, a painful swallow and a period of several days' misery, usually with absence from school, all of which are typical of true bacterial tonsillitis. OSA (see Chapter 16) is the other common indication for tonsillectomy.

Surgical techniques vary. The traditional approach is 'cold steel dissection' with ties or diathermy haemostasis, but a variety of 'hot' techniques including coblation™ (controlled ablation) have become popular in recent years. These have the advantage of reduced perioperative bleeding and permit 'intracapsular' tonsillectomy so that the pharyngeal muscles are not breached, leading to much less postoperative pain and discomfort.

Surgery is often carried out on a day-case basis, with minimal risk of complications. Some degree of pain and discomfort is probably inevitable, easily managed with simple analgesics, but bleeding and airway obstruction are now much less common. Bleeding of such severity as to warrant return to theatre in the immediate postoperative period (primary haemorrhage) can occur in as many as 2% of cases and is a surgical emergency. A later bleed (secondary haemorrhage) is often thought to be due to infection. Quoted rates vary up to over 10% depending on the criteria use to define a 'secondary bleed'.

ADENOIDS

The adenoids are rudimentary at birth but enlarge to occupy a substantial part of the nasopharynx between the ages of about 2 and 7 years. Adenoids can obstruct the nasopharyngeal airway and the orifices of the Eustachian tube, contributing respectively to OSA and OME. There has been increasing focus in recent years on the role of the adenoids as a reservoir of chronic infection. 'Biofilms' are aggregates of bacteria in a complex mucopolysaccharide matrix which is resistant to conventional antimicrobial therapy and may contribute to recurrent infections in the nose, sinuses and middle ear. Adenoidectomy – often in association with an intervention such as tonsillectomy (typically for OSA) or insertion of grommets – is a common ORL procedure in children. Indications include OSA, OME and persistent rhinitis that has been resistant to medical therapy. Blind curettage with a sharp blade has been the traditional technique, but ORL specialists are increasingly moving towards surgery under direct vision (coblation and suction diathermy) using an endoscope and a screen/monitor, permitting much more accurate and thorough removal of tissue. The main complication of adenoidectomy is bleeding. *Velopharyngeal insufficiency,* characterised by escape of air from the nasal cavity during phonation (rhinolalia aperta), is often noted in the weeks and months following surgery but is usually temporary. Persistent cases can be troublesome and, very occasionally, warrant corrective pharyngeal or palatal surgery.

'Grisel's syndrome' is postoperative hypermobility of the neck, causing pain and impaired rotation with the potential for injury to the cervical spinal cord in extreme cases. It was considered a complication of adenotonsillectomy, particularly in children with Down syndrome due to pre-existing laxity of the ligaments that support the atlantoaxial joint. It is now accepted that this can occur following any surgery that involves manipulation of the neck and, while children with Down syndrome are at increased risk, it is important that surgeons and theatre personnel exercise great care when manipulating any child's neck during anaesthesia and surgery.

TONGUE TIE

The lingual frenulum connects the undersurface of the tongue with the floor of the mouth. If it is unusually short or tight (anklyoglossia), tongue movement may be restricted (**Figure 15.2**). Parents will notice a notch at the tip of the tongue when the child protrudes the tongue, and the newborn baby may have difficulty with breastfeeding due to being unable to 'latch'. If the frenulum is divided in the first few days of life, feeding can be greatly improved. In older children, the adverse effects of tongue tie are less certain. Whether a severe tongue tie can interfere with the development of speech is uncertain, but many children and parents will present for treatment due to perceived speech difficulties or difficulty with, for example, playing wind instruments, or with aesthetic concerns.

Treatment in most cases involves simple division of the frenulum, with, in rare cases where the tissue is

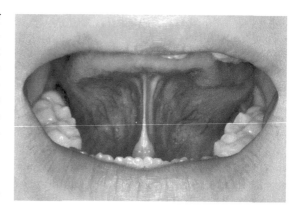

Figure 15.2 Tongue tie.

especially thickened and fixed, a frenuloplasty with a Z-plasty type repair. Newborns will tolerate a frenulotomy without the need for anaesthesia, but older children will need a general anaesthetic.

MACROGLOSSIA

Enlargement of the tongue such that it protrudes beyond the incisors at rest is termed 'macroglossia' (**Figure 15.3**). True enlargement is less common than 'pseudomacroglossia', i.e. the tongue size is normal but protrusion is due to poor muscle control or a relatively small oral cavity. This occurs in some cases of cerebral palsy and in Down syndrome. True macroglossia may be due to hypertrophy of the tongue musculature ('primary' macroglossia, e.g. *Beckwith–Wiedemann* syndrome, *congenital hypothyroidism*), or infiltration of the tongue (secondary macroglossia, e.g. lymphangioma, mucopolysaccharidosis). Symptoms include drooling, ulceration of exposed mucosa, speech difficulties, airway obstruction and aesthetic concerns.

Most children with macroglossia will be under the care of a paediatrician, who will supervise the necessary investigations, but the ORL team may be asked to help if treatment is needed. The child may need airway support with a Guedel airway or, in severe

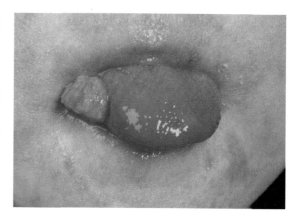

Figure 15.3 Macroglossia. A pyogenic granuloma has developed on the exposed mucosa.

cases, a tracheostomy. Surgical reduction of the tongue (partial glossectomy) is usually undertaken in a specialist centre by an experienced team with appropriate back-up facilities including a PICU.

CLEFT LIP AND PALATE

Cleft of the lip and/or palate occurs in about 1 in 700 births. Most cases are of unknown aetiology, but factors that increase the risk include maternal use of some anticonvulsant agents (phenobarbital, phenytoin), maternal use of alcohol and tobacco, and steroids. Dedicated multidisciplinary teams including a cleft surgeon, orthodontist, speech and language therapist, and otolaryngologist are now well established and offer optimum care for these children and their families. ORL issues include otitis media, nasal deformity with functional and aesthetic issues, and airway obstruction.

Otitis media is so prevalent in children with cleft palate as to be almost universal. The ORL and audiology specialist will need to monitor hearing and treat OME and retraction pockets as needed. Most ORL specialists who look after children with cleft palate will advise caution regarding the use of tympanostomy tubes, as the OME issues may be prolonged and amplification using hearing aids may be more appropriate.

Some conditions (e.g. *Pierre Robin sequence*, see Chapter 3) are associated with significant airway obstruction. A nasopharyngeal airway (NPA) may tide things over until the child is able to manage without airway support. Some children with cleft palate will have other deformities of the head and neck which necessitate a tracheostomy (see Chapter 25).

A variety of palatal clefting of particular importance to ORL is the 'submucous cleft palate'. There is no 'gap' in the mucosa of the palate, but a diastasis of the underlying muscles sometimes with a bifid uvula (**Figure 15.4**), a notch in the hard palate and a visible furrow along the midline of the soft palate (Calnan's triad). Treatment is rarely needed, but extreme caution needs to be taken if adenoidectomy is contemplated, as the adenoids may provide useful bulk behind the soft palate to aid closure during phonation, and overenthusiastic adenoidectomy can cause velopharyngeal insufficiency.

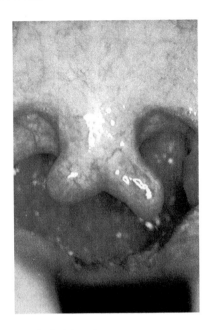

Figure 15.4 Bifid uvula.

KEY POINTS

- Tonsillitis is usually viral. Antibiotics are not always needed.
- Asymmetry of the size of the tonsils is common and causes much parental anxiety, but it is rarely due to serious pathology. The size of the tonsils fluctuates. Carefully assess each case clinically.
- Tongue tie may interfere with breastfeeding in the newborn. Make sure the baby is referred and treated early if there are any concerns. Tongue tie in older children is rarely problematic and won't usually need surgery. The effect on speech is very uncertain.

FURTHER READING

ENT UK Guidelines. Available at: https://www.entuk.org/resources/155/ent_uk_tonsillectomy_commissioning_guide (accessed 25 January 2022).

Mitchell RB, Archer SM, MD, Ishman SL, Rosenfeld RM et al. Clinical Practice Guideline: Tonsillectomy in children (update)–Executive summary. *Otolaryngol Head Neck Surg.* 2019;160(2):187–205. doi: 10.1177/0194599818807917.

Patel S, Burgess A. Paediatric Pathways: Tonsillitis and peritonsillar abscess (quinsy) pathway for children presenting to hospital. Available at: https://bsac.org.uk/paediatricpathways/tonsillitis-quinsy.php (accessed 25 January 2022).

16

OBSTRUCTIVE
SLEEP APNOEA

INTRODUCTION

The spectrum of sleep-disordered breathing (SDB) ranges from simple snoring to severe obstructive sleep apnoea (OSA). The characteristic feature of OSA is cessation of breathing (apnoea) due to partial or complete upper airway obstruction during sleep for periods long enough and frequent enough to cause hypoxaemia. Prevalence is between 2% and 5% of children, primarily up to the age of about 5 years. OSA is especially common in children with Down sundrome (trisomy 21), in obese children (although the relationship is not nearly as direct as it is in adults, and most children with OSA are of normal weight), in children with neurological conditions such as cerebral palsy and in children with craniofacial anomalies.

PATHOPHYSIOLOGY

Good quality sleep in children is essential for normal growth and development. Rapid eye movement (REM) sleep is especially disturbed in OSA with the potential for significant long-term adverse consequences for the child's health. Failure to thrive, ventricular hypertrophy, systemic and pulmonary hypertension, and cor-pulmonale are all recognised long-term consequences of untreated OSA. More immediate effects include daytime sleepiness, irritability, hyperactivity, cognitive dysfunction and behavioural issues.

CLINICAL PRESENTATION

The typical presentation is with snoring, often very noisy and prolonged, leading to disturbed sleep for the child and family. Parents will describe apnoeic episodes during which the child stops breathing, usually while struggling to get air into the respiratory system as evidenced by recession of the chest in younger children, unusual postures, 'tossing and turning' in the bed followed by an arousal response when the child 'wakes themselves up' and recommences normal breathing. These apnoeic spells are alarming for parents who worry that the child may go on to prolonged apnoea, but the hypoxia brought about by an apnoeic episode precipitates a pronounced response in the respiratory centre ('arousal')

DOI: 10.1201/9780429019128-16

so that oxygen saturation is restored. Daytime symptoms such as tiredness, irritability and poor attention are common, and the child will often show features of airway obstruction during the day (e.g. mouth-breathing). The adverse effects on the quality of life of both child and family are considerable and usually greatly improve following adenotonsillectomy.

INVESTIGATIONS

Various parental questionnaires have been used to screen for OSA, and it is likely that the disorder is even more common than the current referral pattern would suggest, i.e. many children have undiagnosed OSA. Parents will often come to the ORL clinic with a mobile-phone video clip showing the child during sleep, and this can be really helpful to demonstrate the apnoeic spells and the attempts to breathe against resistance. Definitive diagnosis of OSA requires measurement of the number of 'apnoeas' (complete cessation of airflow) and 'hypopnoeas' (reduction in airflow) during a defined period – typically an hour – i.e. the apnoea/hypopnoea index (AHI). 'Mild' OSA is associated with an AHI of up to 5, with an AHI of greater than 5 classified as moderate to severe. The 'gold standard' diagnostic tool is polysomnography (PSG), a full 'sleep study' to include electroencephalography, electromyography to measure chest wall movement, nasal flow measurement and a record of respiratory effort in addition to oxygen saturation. Very few units have the capacity or resources for PSG, hence the reliance on overnight pulse oximetry, which can be recorded at home on a portable device.

Pulse oximetry is widely used as a screening tool and diagnostic modality and to 'triage' patients who may need more intensive perioperative care, including overnight stay or even a short stay in a high-dependency unit (HDU). Oxygen desaturation is considered a 'proxy' measurement to record apnoea or hypopnoea but there are limitations and, in practice, the diagnosis of OSA is usually made clinically, based on a typical history often (but by no means always) in a child with obvious adeno-tonsillar enlargement (**Figure 16.1**).

Some children – especially children with a background neurological condition such as cerebral palsy – will

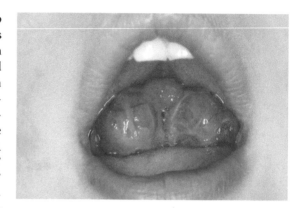

Figure 16.1 Large obstructing tonsils.

have 'central' apnoea, where the apnoeic spells are due not to obstruction but to an abnormal pattern of arousal in the respiratory centre. SDB can, of course, be a mixture of OSA and central apnoea. More sophisticated investigations, including PSG or a variant of PSG depending on local investigative facilities, may be needed in these children.

There is increasing interest in *drug-induced sleep endoscopy* (DISE). The child is given a titrated dose of an anaesthetic agent (usually propofol) and the surgeon passes a flexible endoscope to observe the movements of the tongue, palate and pharyngeal muscles. The technique is especially helpful in children who have had adenotonsillectomy but present with residual symptoms. Adenoidal remnants, tongue base or pharyngeal wall prolapse and, in some cases, laryngomalacia may be picked up in this way.

A few centres use dynamic MRI to study the movement of various parts of the pharynx and upper airway during respiration. This requires general anaesthesia and is still undergoing evaluation.

The great majority of children with OSA will improve following adenotonsillectomy. New techniques of intracapsular tonsillectomy ('tonsillotomy'), including the use of the Coblator™, have led to less intraoperative bleeding and a reduced need for opiate analgesia and facilitated same-day surgery in many cases. Local arrangements vary according to facilities, the experience of the clinical team, parental expectation and resources. In the UK, children over the age of 2 years or with a weight of 12 kg are suitable for surgery in their local hospital without the need for HDU facilities, and children of 1 year and over (corresponding weight 10 kg) can have their surgery locally if there is access to an HDU. Children with significant comorbidity are best referred to a specialist centre where PICU and support services are available (**Box 16.1**).

Box 16.1 Risk factors in the management of OSA

- Severe cerebral palsy
- Achondroplasia
- Neuromuscular disorders (moderately or severely affected)
- Significant craniofacial anomalies
- Mucopolysaccharidosis
- Significant comorbidity (e.g. complex or uncorrected congenital heart disease, home oxygen, severe cystic fibrosis)
- When onsite support from tertiary medical specialties is needed (e.g. metabolic, haematology)

Adenotonsillectomy in OSA is associated with substantial improvements in quality-of-life measurements. Some children with significant comorbidities,

with mixed (central and obstructive) apnoeas and who have severe OSA that has not responded to surgery may need treatment with continuous positive airway pressure (CPAP). Very occasionally, a nasopharyngeal airway, surgery to the craniofacial skeleton or even a tracheostomy will have to be considered.

KEY POINTS

- OSA has a significant effect on the quality of life of both the child and family.
- Most children improve greatly following adenotonsillectomy.

FURTHER READING

Benedek P, Balakrishnan K, Cunningham MJ, Friedman NR et al. International Pediatric Otolaryngology Group (IPOG) consensus on the diagnosis and management of pediatric obstructive sleep apnea (OSA). *Int J Pediatr Otorhinolaryngol.* 2020;138:110276. doi: 10.1016/j.ijporl.2020.110276.

Marcus CL, Moore RH, Rosen CL, Giordani B et al. A randomized trial of adenotonsillectomy for childhood sleep apnea. *N Engl J Med.* 2013;368(25):2366–76. doi: 10.1056/NEJMoa1215881.

Narayanasamy S, Kidambi SS, Mahmoud M, Subramanyam R. Pediatric sleep disordered breathing: a narrative review. *Pediatric Medicine* vol. 2 (October 2019). Available at: https://pm.amegroups.com/article/view/5050/html (accessed 25 January 2022).

17 CONGENITAL NASAL DISORDERS

INTRODUCTION

Nasal obstruction in the newborn is an emergency requiring urgent referral and treatment. Babies are obligate nasal breathers, and any obstruction to nasal airflow at birth will cause severe hypoxaemia, only relieved when the baby breathes through the mouth.

EMBRYOLOGY OF THE NOSE

The nose and sinuses develop from the primitive foregut. Two epithelial elevations (nasal placodes) appear at about the fourth intrauterine week. They fuse to form the lateral nasal walls and the midline septum extends dorsally to separate the nose into the two nasal cavities, each closed behind by the bucconasal membrane. A persistent bucconasal membrane presents as *choanal atresia*.

Partial or complete agenesis of the nose (*arrhinia*) has been described and is a neonatal emergency requiring immediate airway support (a Guedel airway followed in many cases by a tracheostomy).

The developing nose is closely related to the primitive forebrain, from which it becomes separated by the bony structures of the anterior skull base, including the cribriform plate. The developing brain may herniate into the nasal cavity, giving rise to a meningocoele or encephalocoele, which can then present as a nasal mass.

CHOANAL ATRESIA

Failure of canalisation of the posterior nasal apertures (choanae) may be bony, membranous or mixed. It is usually bilateral and presents at birth with 'cyclical cyanosis'. The baby has complete nasal obstruction and becomes hypoxaemic except during mouth breathing, hence it becomes almost impossible to feed the child. If the diagnosis is suspected, the midwife or neonatologist will try to gently pass a small suction catheter from the anterior nares into the nasopharynx. If it fails to pass bilaterally, consider the diagnosis of choanal atresia. A good confirmatory test is to place a cold stainless-steel spatula or mirror just under the baby's anterior nares during a breath cycle to test for misting and condensation (mirror test).

DOI: 10.1201/9780429019128-17

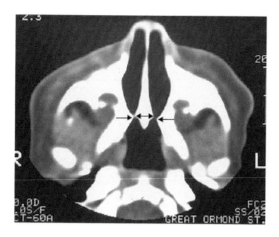

Figure 17.1 CT scan showing choanal stenosis (arrowed).

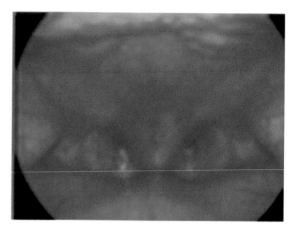

Figure 17.2 The nasal choanae (endoscopic view, 120° telescope).

Neonatal rhinitis and obstruction of the nose due to secretions is commoner than choanal atresia and in many suspected cases no atresia is found.

The first step in management is to secure a safe airway. A Guedel tube in the oral cavity may suffice to enable safe transfer to a paediatric centre, but ET intubation may be needed, especially as many of these children have associated medical conditions.

Imaging (CT scanning) helps to confirm the diagnosis and plan definitive treatment (**Figure 17.1**). A little nasal suction and a few drops of a decongestant (e.g. 0.5% ephedrine) help to clear the nares and make for a more helpful image. Definitive treatment is surgical and should be undertaken as quickly as the baby is stable. Delay may compromise breastfeeding in particular and, if immediate treatment is not possible, a nasogastric tube is best.

There are a variety of surgical techniques for repair. Older methods relied on an open transpalatal approach, but improved modern endoscopes – especially the 120-degree telescope which permits a highly

detailed view of the posterior nares on a monitor (**Figure 17.2**) to facilitate trans-nasal surgery under vision – is more popular.

When the posterior nasal apertures have been established – usually with serial bougie dilatation – bone and soft tissue including in the region of the thickened vomer may be removed with bone forceps and a microdebrider to enlarge the orifices and fashion good-sized choanae. Some surgeons use postoperative stents, but many prefer not to. The baby can soon feed but will need careful follow-up as recurrent stenosis is not uncommon.

In some children, choanal atresia is an isolated anomaly, but it may be associated with a series of linked congenital defects – CHARGE association. Features may include some or all of: **c**oloboma, **h**eart anomalies, **a**tresia of the choanae, **r**enal anomalies, **g**enital hypoplasia, **e**ar anomalies, and it is important that babies are screened by a paediatrician.

Unilateral choanal atresia is much less common and does not usually present until later, usually with unexplained nasal discharge.

PYRIFORM APERTURE STENOSIS

The bony orifices in the midfacial skeleton on either side of the nasal septum that mark the anterior

nares make up the 'pyriform aperture'. Stenosis here is much less common and usually due to excessive prominence of the nasal process of the maxilla. It often mimics choanal atresia but the diagnosis becomes clear on CT scanning.

The early management is the same as for choanal atresia: establish a safe airway, and serial dilatation with decongestant drops and saline irrigation may tide things over and avoid the need for surgery.

Definitive repair, if needed, is more challenging and may require an open rhinoplasty or midfacial degloving approach. There is an association with sometimes very significant intracranial anomalies such as holoprosencephaly (a defect in the development of the midline intracranial structures) and a single central incisor tooth. Again, paediatric liaison for screening is important.

NASAL ENCEPHALOCOELE

A portion of the developing brain may herniate through the bony skull base and become 'trapped' below the cribriform plate within the nasal cavity. This will present as a nasal mass and persist in the nose, often with acute nasal obstruction in the newborn. An *encephalocoele* contains both meninges and neurological tissue in direct continuity with the intracranial structures (**Figure 17.3**). A *meningocoele* is similar but contains no neurological tissue, just the meninges and cerebrospinal fluid. A *glioma* contains nerve tissue (glial cells, usually with fibrous and vascular tissue) but is discrete from the intracranial contents, i.e. it has become 'pinched off'. *Glial heterotopia* refers to the presence of a mass of such tissue in an aberrant site, i.e. the nasal cavity or the nasopharynx where it may have migrated some distance from its intracranial origin.

Detailed and skilled imaging is essential in the management of these lesions. Their possible connection to intracranial structures leaves the child at risk of catastrophic intracranial sepsis, especially in the case of injudicious surgery or biopsy. MRI is most suitable if available and will demonstrate intracranial connection if present. Treatment is surgical. Gliomas may be removed trans-nasally, but encephalocoeles and meningocoeles, especially if large, will often need an open combined ORL and neurosurgical approach.

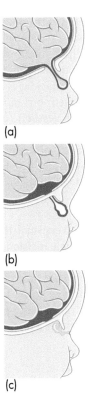

(a)

(b)

(c)

Figure 17.3 Congenital nasal masses. (a) Encephalocoele. Neural tissue projects into the nasal cavity. (b) Meningocoele. Meninges with contained CSF projects into the nasal cavity. (c) Glioma. Neural tissue in the nasal cavity but no remaining connection to the cranial cavity.

A variety of cysts – derived from embryonic tissue – can present in and around the nasal structures in the newborn.

▋ Dermoid cyst

The commonest congenital nasal mass is a dermoid cyst . This is typically a smooth midline swelling on the dorsum of the nose under the skin. There may be an external 'punctum'. It is thought to result from inclusion of epithelial cells along lines of fusion, hence the tendency for it to occur in the midline. The cyst contains thick, often viscous fluid, with ectodermal and mesodermal components, sometimes including skin appendages and hair follicles. It may become infected, but more often the parents will present with aesthetic concerns. Careful evaluation including detailed imaging is essential, not least to exclude an intracranial connection as these lesions can invaginate deeply into the midline nasal cartilages and beyond, making excision very challenging.

Treatment is surgical. Very small discrete lesions can be removed with a single incision on the nasal dorsum, or endoscopically, but an external rhinoplasty approach can make for a more satisfactory aesthetic result. Larger and more extensive lesions will require liaison with neurosurgical colleagues and may need a frontonasal approach via a forehead incision.

▋ Nasolacrimal duct cysts

Nasolacrimal duct cysts may preset to the ORL clinic with nasal obstruction, or to the eye clinic with epiphora. If they require surgery, a trans-nasal endoscopic approach is usually possible.

▋ Nasoalveolar and nasolabial cysts

Nasoalveolar cysts in the floor of the nose and *nasolabial cysts* along the lateral nasal wall may cause aesthetic concerns. They can usually be removed safely by enucleation, taking care not to leave any epithelial remnants behind.

▋ Odontogenic or dentigerous cysts

Odontogenic (or *dentigerous*) *cysts* occur in association with the development and eruption of the teeth and may occur in the maxillary antrum and the floor of the nose.

▋ Thornwaldt's cyst

Thornwaldt's cyst is a midline usually asymptomatic nasopharyngeal cyst, increasingly found as endoscopic inspection of the nasopharynx (e.g. during adenoidectomy) becomes more commonplace.

▋ Teratoma

Teratoma is a neoplastic cystic lesion containing all three germinal cell layers. It may present as a firm obstructing nasal mass. Very large teratomas may be diagnosed *in utero* and may be associated with maternal polyhydramnios. Investigation is via CT and MRI scanning.

The treatment is surgical, and regular follow-up may be assisted by serial alphafetoprotein measurements.

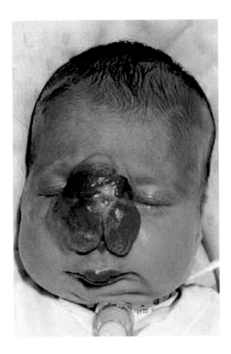

Figure 17.4 Nasal haemangioma.

VASCULAR MALFORMATIONS

Haemangiomas of the head and neck are relatively common, usually cutaneous, and do not always need treatment (**Figure 17.4**). Large proliferating haemangiomas in and around the nose may cause severe airway compromise as well as worrying aesthetic effects. Medical treatment is with propranolol, but in highly aggressive lesions – especially if they encroach on the orbit and threaten vision – mitomycin C can be considered.

THE NASAL SEPTUM

Some degree of deviation of the nasal septum is so common as to be normal. This may be due to compression of the facial skeleton at delivery. Unless there is gross cosmetic deformity or severe airway obstruction, nasal septal surgery is usually discouraged before the mid to late teens due to the risk of a poor aesthetic result ('saddle nose'). Prominent blood vessels on the nasal septum (Little's area or Kiesselbach's plexus) can cause nosebleeds (epistaxis) but in children a dilated vein just under the septal mucosa can be to blame. This usually responds well to silver nitrate cautery.

KEY POINTS

- Neonatal rhinitis is much more common than choanal atresia.
- Early correction of choanal atresia is important to enable the baby to feed.
- Avoid biopsy or instrumentation of congenital nasal masses until you have good quality imaging. Many congenital nasal masses have an intracranial connection.

FURTHER READING

Moreddu E, Rizzi M, Adil E, Balakrishnan K et al. International Pediatric Otolaryngology Group (IPOG) consensus recommendations: Diagnosis, pre-operative, operative and post-operative pediatric choanal atresia care. *Int J Pediatr Otorhinolaryngol.* 2019;123:151–5. doi: 10.1016/j.ijporl.2019.05.010.

ACUTE RHINOSINUSITIS

INTRODUCTION

'Colds', 'sniffles', viral upper respiratory tract infections and nasal discharge are a universal feature of childhood. Children with these conditions are generally looked after by their parents or carers at home and do not usually need medical attention (**Figure 18.1**). As the mucosa of the nose and the

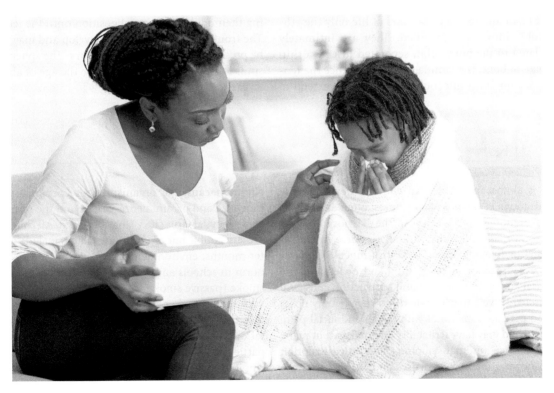

Figure 18.1 Acute rhinosinusitis (ARS) is an almost universal experience in childhood.

DOI: 10.1201/9780429019128-18

paranasal sinuses is one continuous epithelial lining, it is inevitable that rhinitis is accompanied by sinusitis, hence the term 'rhinosinusitis' is preferred to describe inflammation in this region. Given the number of healthcare professionals (paediatricians, family doctors, nurses, etc.) who attend to children with rhinosinusitis and the ubiquity and variety of the presentations treated, the definitions, terminology and therapeutic recommendations can be confusing. The European Position Paper on Rhinosinusitis and Nasal Polyps (EPOS) clarifies some of these issues and contains considered evidence-based guidelines for the diagnosis and management of rhinosinusitis, including acute rhinosinusitis (ARS), in both adults and children (**Box 18.1**).

> ### Box 18.1 Acute rhinosinusitis in children
>
> ARS in children is defined as: sudden onset of two or more of the symptoms:
>
> - nasal blockage/obstruction/congestion
> - discoloured nasal discharge
> - cough (daytime and night-time)
>
> for <12 weeks; with symptom-free intervals if the problem is recurrent; with validation by telephone or interview.
>
> *Source*: European Position Paper on Rhinosinusitis and Nasal Polyps 2020 (EPOS2020), p. 2.

ANATOMICAL CONSIDERATIONS

The configuration and pneumatisation of the sinuses in children markedly differ from those of the adult. At birth and in the early years of life only the ethmoid sinuses are air-filled. They are intimately related to the bony orbit, separated just by a thin plate of bone, the lamina papyracea, hence the tendency for sinus infections in children to extend to the orbit (orbital cellulitis, see Chapter 5). The maxillary sinuses are rudimentary at birth, not reaching their adult volume and position until the teens. The frontal sinus is the last to develop and may not be present before the age of 10 years. The sphenoid sinus is rarely pneumatised before the age of about 5 years.

PATHOPHYSIOLOGY

It is almost inevitable that children develop acute infections of the nose and sinuses, often as many as ten or more episodes in a year. The diagnosis is nearly always made clinically without recourse to endoscopy or imaging. There is a brisk mucosal inflammatory reaction with swelling and oedema of the nasal and sinus mucosa, nasal obstruction and nasal discharge. Features include rhinorrhea (runny nose) and pyrexia, sometimes with cough and facial pain. The child may have irritability and malaise but many experience minimal symptoms and little disruption to normal life. Adenoviruses and rhinoviruses are common causative organisms, but coronaviruses, influenza and parainfluenza viruses and the respiratory syncytial virus (RSV) may be found. All children are susceptible but predisposing factors include winter months, environmental exposure such as is the norm in schools and nurseries, exposure to tobacco smoke (passive smoking) and immunodeficiency. A very small number of children have ciliary motility disorders, and anatomical factors such as nasal septal deviation and/or (dental) sepsis may predispose particularly to bacterial infection. The role of allergic rhinitis (AR) is unclear.

Care pathways for acute rhinusitis (ARS)

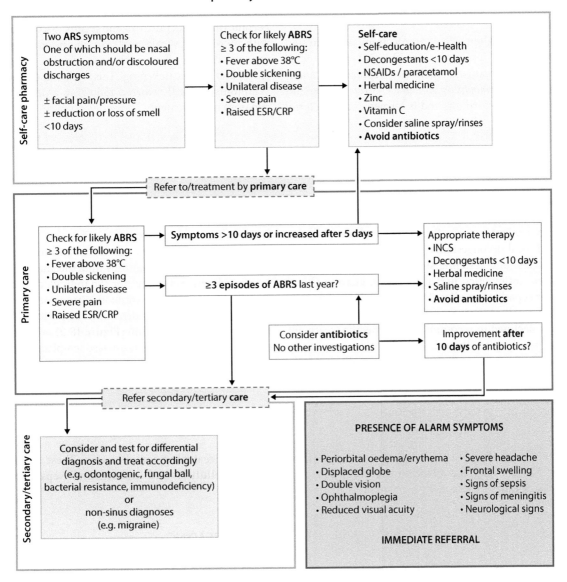

Figure 18.2 EPOS management algorithm for ARS.

OUTCOMES

The infection is generally self-limiting and resolves with or without treatment. If symptoms worsen after 5 days, or persist for 10 days or more, the EPOS guidelines suggest the term 'post-viral ARS'. Some children are prone to repeated episodes – more than four per annum – *recurrent acute rhinosinusitis* (*RARS*). This may be confused with AR and with bronchial asthma. Whether RARS is a causative factor in the development of bronchial asthma is unclear.

In a few children, the viral infection is complicated by bacterial superinfection. This is typically with pyogenic organisms such as *Streptococcus pneumoniae, Haemophilus influenzae, Strep. Milleri* and *Moraxella catarrhalis* and is termed *acute bacterial rhinosinusitis (ABRS)*. Clinically, this presents as a change in the nature of the rhinorrhea, which may become thickened, purulent and greatly discoloured, with increased pyrexia and systemic upset, raised inflammatory markers such as C-reactive protein (CRP) and 'double sickening'. This is when the child's symptoms suddenly worsen following a period of apparent improvement.

MANAGEMENT

Treatment is largely supportive and symptomatic. Multiple therapeutic interventions have been used and evaluated for ARS. These include systemic and local decongestants, intranasal corticosteroids (INCSs) and systemic steroids, antibiotics, probiotics, antipyretics, herbal remedies, vitamin C and homeopathic remedies. The evidential base for more or less all of these is at best uncertain, and EPOS has declined to recommend any specific treatment for routine use. The role of antibiotics is especially contentious. The effect, if any, is small, and only applicable if there is a true bacterial infection. The most appropriate antibiotics in most situations are amoxycillin or a cephalosporin. This must be balanced against the alarming rise in antimicrobial resistance in all communities and the morbidity associated with antibiotics for the individual child. Despite these concerns, antibiotics are widely used in practice and are often demanded by parents. The EPOS guidelines/algorithm (**Figure 18.2**) presents a considered and well evidence-based template for use in primary and secondary care.

COMPLICATIONS

Although usually no more than a nuisance, albeit with a considerable effect on the child and parents' quality of life, ARS can give rise to serious and life-threatening complications. These include orbital cellulitis and intracranial sepsis (see Chapter 5).

KEY POINTS

- Upper respiratory tract infections and nasal discharge are universal features of childhood.
- The European Position Paper on Rhinosinusitis and Nasal Polyps (EPOS) contains considered evidence-based guidelines for the diagnosis and management of ARS.
- Antibiotics are only required if there is a true bacterial infection.

FURTHER READING

Dennison SH, Hertting O, Bennet R, Eriksson M et al. A Swedish population-based study of complications due to acute rhinosinusitis in children 5–18 years old. *Int J Pediatr Otorhinolaryngol.* 2021;150:110866. doi: 10.1016/j.ijporl.2021.110866.

Fokkens WJ, Lund VJ, Hopkins C, Hellings PW et al. European Position Paper on Rhinosinusitis and Nasal Polyps 2020 (EPOS2020). *Rhinology* 2020;58(Suppl S29):1–464. doi: 10.4193/Rhin20.600. Available at: https://epos2020.com/Documents/supplement_29.pdf (accessed 26 January 2022).

19

CHRONIC RHINOSINUSITIS

INTRODUCTION

Acute rhinosinusitis usually resolves but a small proportion of children will go on to have persistent symptoms. Rhinosinusitis persisting beyond 12 weeks is referred to as *chronic rhinosinusitis* (*CRS*). This is characterised by rhinorrhea and nasal obstruction (**Box 19.1**) and is an important cause of long-term morbidity in children.

PATHOPHYSIOLOGY

CRS is primarily an infective condition, but there is some overlap with AR and the two may coexist. Pyogenic organisms – *Streptococcus pneumoniae, Haemophilus influenzae, Moraxella catarrhalis* – elicit a chronic inflammatory reaction causing oedema and exudation of the nasal mucosa. Clinically, the mucosa is suffused and swollen, especially in the region of the inferior and middle turbinates, causing obstruction of the sinus ostia. The sinus epithelium becomes engorged, sometimes with a purulent discharge, which causes congestion and facial pain. 'Biofilms' are now thought to play an important role. These are aggregates of bacteria, secretions and host inflammatory cells in a complex mucopolysaccharide matrix which adheres to mucosal surfaces and is relatively resistant to both host defences and antimicrobial therapy. The biofilm forms a reservoir of continuing infection and, periodically, sheds bacteria which can migrate and

> ### Box 19.1 Definition of chronic rhinosinusitis in children
>
> Chronic rhinosinusitis (with or without nasal polyps) in children is defined as: the presence of two or more symptoms one of which should be either nasal blockage / obstruction / congestion or nasal discharge (anterior/posterior nasal drip):
>
> - ± facial pain/pressure
> - ± cough
>
> for ≥12 weeks; with validation by telephone or interview.
>
> *Source*: European Position Paper on Rhinosinusitis and Nasal Polyps 2020 (EPOS 2020), p. 3.

DOI: 10.1201/9780429019128-19

establish further biofilms at adjacent sites. Biofilms on both the nasal mucosa and adenoids may contribute to CRS, making elimination of the infecting organisms very difficult.

CLINICAL FEATURES

Prolonged nasal congestion and discharge are the dominant symptoms. Examination will show nasal obstruction, often a mucopurulent exudate (**Figure 19.1**), congestion and swelling of the mucosa – particularly marked in the region of the middle turbinates – and sometimes crusting and exudation.

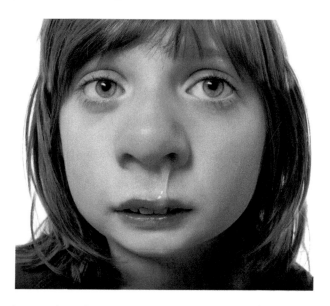

Figure 19.1 Nasal discharge, often of a mucopurulent exudate, is a dominant symptom of CRS.

INVESTIGATIONS

CRS is a clinical diagnosis, and few children need complex investigations. Thorough nasendoscopy can be undertaken in the ORL clinic. Most children have no underlying conditions, but some will have anatomical abnormalities of the nose (e.g. severe septal deformity) or, in very rare cases, an undiagnosed unilateral choanal atresia. A small number of children have immunodeficiency, and ORL specialists need to be alert to the possibility that primary ciliary dyskinesia (PCD) or cystic fibrosis (CF) can present to the ENT clinic. Arrange appropriate investigations if you are suspicious; for example, consider a 'sweat test' or genetic testing to exclude CF particularly if the child has nasal polyps. If there is diagnostic uncertainty or coexisting AR, skin tests may be helpful. Imaging (CT scanning) will show extensive mucosal disease and may demonstrate an antrochoanal polyp or an unexpected nasal mass.

TREATMENT

Treatment of CRS is primarily medical. Saline nasal irrigation is safe and effective and may be well tolerated by some children. The evidence base for most pharmacological interventions in children is weak, but INCSs are usually recommended, certainly before contemplating any surgical treatment. EPOS guidelines recommend that surgery should only be considered following 'appropriate medical treatment' (AMT), and despite the poor evidence base to support the use of antibiotics, most ORL specialists will recommend a course of antibiotics before considering surgery.

SURGERY

There is good evidence to support adenoidectomy for recalcitrant CRS, perhaps because the adenoids act as a reservoir of continuous infection. Maxillary antral lavage has been widely used in the past and is often combined with adenoidectomy. The exact role of functional endoscopic sinus surgery (FESS) is not fully established, but it is frequently used with some evidence of symptomatic improvement. Middle meatal antrostomy and limited removal of diseased mucosa rather than extensive exenteration of the paranasal sinuses is probably all that is needed. Turbinate reduction surgery is often offered as a last resort to improve severe nasal obstruction, but the effect, if any, tends to be short-lived.

FURTHER READING

Fokkens WJ, Lund VJ, Hopkins C, Hellings PW et al. European Position Paper on Rhinosinusitis and Nasal Polyps 2020 (EPOS2020). *Rhinology.* 2020;58(Suppl S29):1–464. doi: 10.4193/Rhin20.600. Available at: https://epos2020.com/Documents/supplement_29.pdf (accessed 26 January 2022).

KEY POINTS

- CRS is an important cause of long-term morbidity in children.
- 'Biofilms' on the nasal mucosa and adenoids may contribute to CRS, making elimination of the infecting organisms very difficult.
- Treatment is primarily medical with surgery reserved for cases that have failed to respond to intensive pharmaco-therapy.

20 ALLERGIC RHINOSINUSITIS

INTRODUCTION

Allergic rhinosinusitis (AR) is becoming increasingly common with a prevalence varying between 10% and 25% in children. It causes severe adverse effects on the quality of life of both child and family, and it is now apparent that effective recognition and management not only improve symptoms but help to control concomitant bronchial asthma.

PATHOGENESIS

AR is an inflammatory condition caused by the cellular response to an allergen to which the child has earlier been exposed. It is mediated by immunoglobulin E (IgE) which binds to receptor cells – 'mast cells' – in the host. The nasal mucosa is especially sensitive but the pharynx, the oral cavity and particularly the conjunctival mucosa are frequently involved, such that the term AR is now best thought of as *allergic rhinoconjunctivitis*. Degranulation of these cells releases a variety of inflammatory mediators such as histamine, leukotriene C4 and others which cause swelling, oedema and hypersensitivity of the mucosa. The typical allergens at play in children are the house dust mite, grass and tree pollens, moulds and spores, and animal (pet) dander. There is a strong genetic component to the aetiology of AR. It is more common in western populations and, while the exact reasons for this are unknown, smaller family size, earlier exposure to environmental pollutants and reduced exposure to community infections may be some of the factors at play.

CLINICAL FEATURES

The dominant symptoms in most children are nasal discharge (usually a thin watery rhinorrhoea), nasal obstruction, sneezing and itching. Swelling and itching of the eyelids due to conjunctivitis are more common than realised and should be enquired about. Some children will experience itching and discomfort in the palate and the pharynx, with symptoms worsening

DOI: 10.1201/9780429019128-20

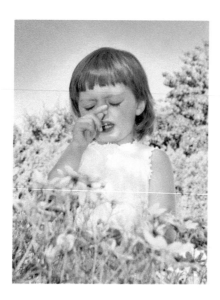

Figure 20.1 Hay fever.

during periods of exposure to the allergen, such as to pollens and grasses in the spring and summer (hay fever, **Figure 20.1**). The effects on quality of life may be very considerable, with reduced school attendance and interference with sport, leisure and exercise.

DIAGNOSIS AND INVESTIGATIONS

AR is typically managed by family doctors and the diagnosis is clinical, with little recourse to endoscopy or investigations. The history is key and, on examination, the nasal mucosa may be moist, swollen, erythematous or sometimes pale with swelling of the inferior and middle turbinates. If the child is seen in an ORL clinic, nasendoscopy will show further evidence of boggy oedematous nasal mucosa, and skin tests to identify specific allergens are often considered. These take the form of intradermal injection of a series of allergens with observation and measurement of the local reaction (a 'wheal'). Blood tests to measure serum IgE – both total IgE and allergen-specific IgE – are sometimes done but they are less accurate than skin tests. Tests in more specialised clinics include nasal smears to identify eosinophils, 'nasal challenge' to provoke response to a specific allergen, and measurement of nitrous oxide (NO). Imaging is not routinely helpful, but CT scanning may be needed if there is nasal polyposis or suspicion regarding an alternative diagnosis (e.g. antrochoanal polyp).

TREATMENT

Early and appropriate management of AR is essential not only to improve the quality of life of the child and family but because there is increasing evidence that good rhinitis control reduces the risk of the development of bronchial asthma and helps to improve the progress of asthma in children already affected.

Allergen avoidance is the first step in AR management. If the child is allergic to house dust mite, then mattress protectors and acaricides for carpets and soft furnishings can help. Most parents will take measures to reduce exposure to grasses, pollens and pet dander, for example, but eliminating common allergens, including pollens and grasses, is not easy.

Pharmacotherapy usually starts with a systemic or intranasal antihistamine, preferably a non-sedating one such as cetirizine or desloratadine. INCSs give very good symptom control. A spray is usually better tolerated than 'drops' and, while inevitably there is some systemic absorption, this is least with the low bioavailability preparations (e.g. mometasone and fluticasone). Leukotriene receptor antagonists tend to be reserved for more severe disease, and a short course of oral glucocorticoids may be considered for extreme exacerbation of symptoms, for example, if the child needs symptom control during school examinations. Despite the low bioavailability of modern INCSs, there is a concern regarding systemic absorption, and it is important to bear in mind that some INCSs can now be bought without prescription, so parents and children may 'self-medicate'.

Nasal decongestants – local and systemic – are discouraged in children, but are sometimes used for short periods to control severe exacerbations.

Sodium chromoglycate, a 'mast cell stabiliser', can be used as a nasal spray, and oral montelukast, a leukotriene receptor antagonist, may have a place.

'Immunotherapy' has enjoyed increased popularity in recent years. The principle is that controlled exposure to the allergen may bring about desensitisation. Two methods are commonly employed: sublingual immunotherapy (SLIT) and subcutaneous immunotherapy (SCIT). These may be available in a small number of centres and in limited circumstances, but the evidence base for their use in children is currently poor, and there is a risk of anaphylaxis.

Surgery has little to offer in the management of AR, but turbinate reduction techniques have been popular in the past where there is gross turbinate hypertrophy and failure to improve nasal obstruction despite intensive medical therapy.

KEY POINTS

- AR has a very considerable impact on the child's quality of life.
- Good control of AR is an important aspect of the management of bronchial asthma.
- AR is a medical disorder. Surgery has little or no place in management.

FURTHER READING

Cingi C, Muluk NB, Scadding GK. Will every child have allergic rhinitis soon? *Int J Pediatr Otorhinolaryngol.* 2019;118:53–8. doi: 10.1016/j.ijporl.2018.12.019.

Fokkens WJ, Lund VJ, Hopkins C, Hellings PW et al. European Position Paper on Rhinosinusitis and Nasal Polyps 2020 (EPOS2020). *Rhinology.* 2020;58(Suppl S29):1–464. doi: 10.4193/Rhin20.600. Available at: https://epos2020.com/Documents/supplement_29.pdf (accessed 26 January 2022).

21

NON-INFLAMMATORY ACQUIRED SINONASAL DISORDERS

INTRODUCTION

Tumours of the nose and paranasal sinuses in children are uncommon and hence not infrequently missed until they are very advanced.

ANGIOFIBROMA

This is a benign but locally invasive fibrovascular tumour almost exclusive to adolescent boys. There may be a hormonal mechanism to explain this but the exact aetiology is unknown. The tumour arises from the sphenopalatine foramen and extends into the nasal cavity and the nasopharynx, compressing the bony facial skeleton and the skull base. Typical presentations are nasal obstruction and epistaxis. Modern imaging techniques – MRI scanning and CT – will demonstrate the mass and delineate the margins. The MRI appearance is highly characteristic with a pronounced 'blush' (**Figure 21.1**). Angiography is not only diagnostic but may facilitate embolisation and help to control what can be torrential perioperative bleeding if resection is planned.

The treatment is surgical removal, even if the mass is small, as progression is inevitable. Early disease may be amenable to endoscopic removal; larger tumours will require an open approach. This type of surgery tends to be concentrated in a few specialist centres where clinicians have gained experience in a number of techniques such as midfacial degloving, lateral rhinotomy and maxillary osteotomy, sometimes combined with endoscopic clearance.

FIBROUS DYSPLASIA

This is a benign lesion of bone which may affect the craniofacial skeleton causing aesthetic and functional nasal problems. It can be 'monostotic', i.e. in a single bony locus, or 'polyostotic' where it can be

DOI: 10.1201/9780429019128-21

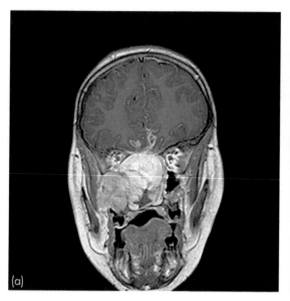
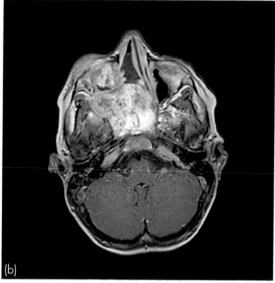

Figure 21.1 MRI appearance of angiofibroma: (a) axial (b) coronal.

present in more than one site, often including one of the long bones (e.g. the femur or tibia). It can occur in older children or young adults, and while not a true neoplasm, the involved bone expands rapidly causing facial deformity, dental malocclusion and encroachment onto the orbit. Diagnosis is by imaging, with a characteristic appearance ('ground glass') on plain X-ray and on CT scanning (**Figure 21.2**). Treatment is conservative as far as possible, but surgery to debulk large lesions may be appropriate for cosmetic reasons. A small number of these children have associated endocrine abnormalities (*McCune–Albright syndrome*) and should be screened by a paediatrician.

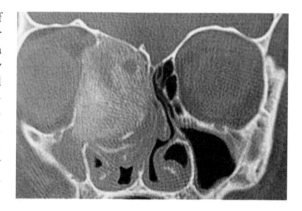

Figure 21.2 CT scan showing fibrous dysplasia of the maxilla.

JUVENILE OSSIFYING FIBROMA

Juvenile ossifying fibroma (JOF) is a true neoplasm which can occur in the craniofacial skeleton. Proptosis, nasal obstruction, epistaxis and facial deformity can all ensue. The radiological appearance is characteristic, showing a radiolucent lesion with variable calcification. Treatment is surgical and complete excision may be very difficult.

MALIGNANCY

Malignant disease in the mucosal or skeletal elements of the nose in childhood is rare, but as a large number of the malignancies that present in children occur in the head and neck, it is important for the ORL specialist to be vigilant. An expanding facial swelling warrants immediate investigations as it is highly suggestive of malignancy (**Figure 21.3**). Arrange imaging and, if necessary, biopsy if suspicious. Lymphoma, Ewing's sarcoma, rhabdomyosarcoma, haemangiopericytoma and nasopharyngeal squamous carcinoma have all been described in the nasal cavity and nasopharynx in children.

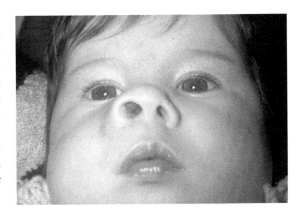

Figure 21.3 An expanding facial swelling, highly suggestive of malignant disease.

NASAL TRAUMA

Despite being highly active and prone to various injuries, young children present relatively infrequently with nasal trauma compared to their young adult counterparts. Check for septal haematomas, associated injuries such as facial fractures and for bony deformity (**Figure 21.4**). The nasal skeleton is relatively soft and pliable in children and deformity requiring surgical correction is not common. If there is a deformity, manipulation under anaesthesia will usually bring about a satisfactory aesthetic result.

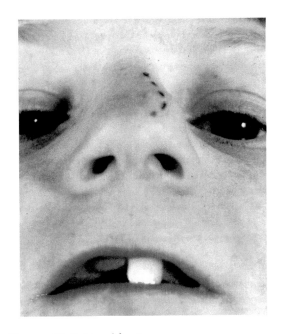

Figure 21.4 Nasal fracture.

KEY POINTS

- Consider flexible nasendoscopy in adolescent boys who present with a nosebleed, especially if bleeds are recurrent or unexpectedly profuse.
- Avoid biopsy of a nasal mass until you have good quality imaging. Bleeding from an angiofibroma may be torrential.

FURTHER READING

Wilson MN, Nuss DW, Zacharia Bek, Snyderman CH. Surgical management of juvenile nasopharyngeal angiofibroma. *Oper Tech Otolaryngol - Head Neck Surg.* 2019;30:22-9.

22 THE OBSTRUCTED AIRWAY

INTRODUCTION

A baby's airway is especially vulnerable to obstruction, given its narrow calibre and the high oxygen needs of the infant. The larynx and trachea in the newborn are less rigid than in an adult or an older child, and hence more susceptible to compression. A small reduction in the diameter of the airway lumen – such as occurs with mucosal swelling in an acute respiratory infection – can have a profound effect.

The infant may struggle hard to breathe, causing immense alarm and distress to parents and healthcare staff alike. Specific causes of airway obstruction in children and their management are covered in the next three chapters. This chapter focuses on the general principles of looking after a child with acute airway obstruction.

CLINICAL PRESENTATION

This will depend on the cause, but some features are constant (**Box 22.1**). A baby with an obstructed airway will be distressed, often demonstrating *tachypnoea*, *recession* of the soft thoracic cage on inspiration, and visible indrawing of the trachea (*tracheal tug*). The child struggles to feed. *Stridor* refers to a high-pitched noise, typically on inspiration, although expiratory stridor can present as well, especially if the obstruction is lower in the airway (e.g. in tracheomalacia). Stridor on inspiration and expiration (*biphasic*) is ominous and suggests severe airway compromise. The low-pitched 'snoring'-type noise associated with pharyngeal airway obstruction is more often referred to as *stertor*, but the terms 'stridor' and 'stertor' are often used imprecisely. The noisy breathing associated with lower airway obstruction (e.g. in bronchial asthma) is usually referred to as '*wheezing*'.

> **Box 22.1 Features of airway obstruction in infants**
>
> - Stridor
> - Tachypnoea
> - 'Tracheal tug'
> - Chest recession
> - Feeding difficulties

DOI: 10.1201/9780429019128-22

With increased work needed for breathing, a child can maintain good oxygen saturations for a considerable period of time, but progressive airway obstruction will tire the child and eventually cause reduced breathing, cyanosis and cardiorespiratory arrest.

Be alert to the 'red flags' to look for in a child with airway obstruction (**Box 22.2**).

> **Box 22.2 'Red flags' in a child with airway obstruction**
>
> - Biphasic stridor
> - Reduced stridor after a prolonged period of struggle ('Beware the quiet child')
> - Cyanosis – a very late sign of impending acidosis and cardiac arrest
> - Bradycardia

EARLY MANAGEMENT

The child may need immediate resuscitation in the acute situation. Healthcare personnel looking after children with potential airway obstruction need to be conversant with the principles of Advanced Paediatric Life Support™ (APLS). The first priority is to ensure the oropharyngeal airway is patent, i.e. check for a foreign body or a prolapsed tongue and apply gentle suction to remove secretions. High-flow oxygen using a re-breathing bag (Ambu-bag™) can buy a little time. Nebulised adrenaline – 2 ml of 1 in 1000 solution in normal saline – may help if there is extensive mucosal swelling or bronchoconstriction, and it is essential to establish good IV access early on. Corticosteroid therapy – dexamethasone 0.4 mg per kg – has been shown to greatly improve the management of children with airway obstruction whatever the cause and should be given early, usually by the subcutaneous route.

Continue to monitor – pulse oximetry, vital signs – and support the airway throughout including, if appropriate, the use of a face mask with hand ventilation. If there is no improvement, the child may need an alternative airway. This is typically via ET intubation or the use of a laryngeal mask if personnel skilled at intubation or the use of the mask are available. If ET intubation is impossible, or if there is a proximal obstruction, a cricothyroidotomy may be considered (**Figure 22.1**). This is very much a procedure used only *in extremis* and should be an absolute last resort, particularly in the very young for whom ET intubation is much preferred.

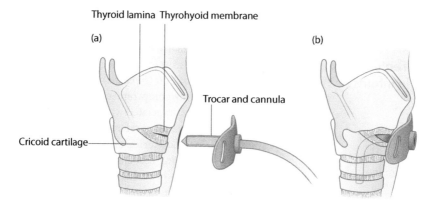

Thyroid lamina Thyrohyoid membrane

(a) (b)

Trocar and cannula

Cricoid cartilage

Figure 22.1 (a,b) Cricothyroid puncture should be used only as a last resort.

ASSESSMENT

Rapid and life-threatening airway obstruction in babies is uncommon, and more often stridor is gradual, intermittent and of varying severity. Once the emergency situation is under control, focus your attention on diagnosis and treatment. Clinical features can help to narrow the diagnosis, and a careful history and examination will dictate the next steps. A rapid onset suggests an acute infection – especially if the child is febrile – or an inhaled foreign body. Hoarseness or an abnormal cry suggests laryngeal pathology such as recurrent respiratory papillomatosis (RRP) in an older child or a cord palsy in a baby. Feeding difficulties and aspiration can occur in tracheo-oesophageal fistula (TOF) or laryngeal cleft, and the birth and neonatal history can alert the clinician to a web, mucosal cysts or laryngotracheal stenosis.

The primary diagnostic technique is *airway endoscopy*. Laryngoscopy is a relatively straightforward outpatient procedure for many children (*flexible awake airway endoscopy*) and should be the first investigative technique if the child will tolerate it.

It is usually easily accomplished in babies by asking the parent to hold the infant on their lap, and in an older child you may be able to secure the child's cooperation.

More thorough endoscopy including rigid *laryngo-tracheobronchoscopy* requires general anaesthesia with the use of Hopkins rod telescopes and a recording monitor. This will usually be undertaken in a centre that has specialist experience in the anaesthetic and surgical management of children with paediatric airway pathology.

Imaging can supplement endoscopy: for example, if tracheal compression is noted at endoscopy, then a CT or MRI scan may demonstrate an abnormal mediastinal vessel. MRI scanning is useful to demonstrate the extent of a haemangioma or a lymphangioma, and contrast studies such as tube oesophagography and bronchography can be useful to demonstrate a TOF or to delineate the extent and severity of tracheobronchomalacia.

DEFINITIVE TREATMENT

Clearly, treatment depends on the cause. The child will often need to be transferred to a specialist centre. Protocols and resources for the transfer of the acutely ill child have greatly improved in recent years and close liaison between the referral centre and the unit where the child presents is important. The child may need ET intubation to facilitate safe transfer (see Chapter 1). In some circumstances, a 'retrieval team' may need to travel to help support the local team and facilitate transport.

FURTHER READING
Advanced Life Support Group (ALSG). Advanced Paediatric Life Support: A practical approach to emergencies, 6th edn. Wiley-Blackwell; 2016.

KEY POINTS

- A small reduction in the diameter of the airway of a young child can have a profound effect.
- Be aware of the common features of airway obstruction in an infant, particularly the 'red flags'.
- Be conversant with the principles of APLS.
- Treatment in a specialist centre may be required.

23

CONGENITAL LARYNGEAL DISEASE

INTRODUCTION

The laryngotracheal structures develop from the primitive foregut. Major anomalies of the air passages often occur in association with oesophageal anomalies, some of which (e.g. tracheal agenesis) are incompatible with survival. Congenital airway pathology will typically, but not always, present as stridor in the newborn. Conditions such as haemangiomas and some cases of laryngotracheal stenosis do not manifest themselves until later.

LARYNGOMALACIA

This is the commonest cause of stridor in infancy. It may present immediately at birth, but it more often becomes problematic in the first few weeks of life as the baby's oxygen needs increase and the child begins to feed. It is characterised by harsh inspiratory stridor, made worse when the child feeds or becomes very active. It usually improves when the child is positioned prone and can become less pronounced when the baby is asleep. Most cases are mild and resolve spontaneously, but severe cases can cause great distress, feeding difficulties, failure to thrive and repeated hospital admissions due to acute exacerbations. The aetiology is not fully understood but is thought to relate to the comparative softness of the baby's laryngeal cartilages such that they are 'drawn in' during respiration. This is easily seen at endoscopy when the epiglottis takes on an 'omega' shape with short aryepiglottic folds and the arytenoid cartilages are rapidly drawn together on inspiration, partially or completely occluding the airway (**Figure 23.1**). There may be redundant and swollen mucosa particularly over the arytenoids, and virtually the whole of the supraglottis can prolapse into the glottis on inspiration.

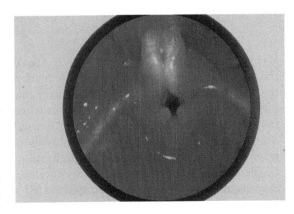

Figure 23.1 Laryngomalacia – endoscopic view of the supraglottis.

DOI: 10.1201/9780429019128-23

Mild cases need no intervention. There is an association with gastro-oesophageal reflux, but the precise relationship is unclear and the role of anti-reflux treatment is uncertain. More severe cases warrant referral to a paediatric ORL clinic where flexible endoscopy will demonstrate the dynamic features and help reassure the parents. Persistent cases, or where there is failure to thrive, diagnostic uncertainty or concern about associated conditions will need admission for rigid airway endoscopy. This is to confirm the diagnosis, exclude any other pathology and, if appropriate, improve the symptoms by surgery. The preferred technique for most paediatric otolaryngologists is an 'aryepiglottoplasty' (**Figure 23.2**). This involves division of the aryepiglottic folds to open the laryngeal introitus, sometimes combined with removal of excessive and redundant mucosa. Excessive tissue removal risks postoperative aspiration, and a conservative approach is preferred.

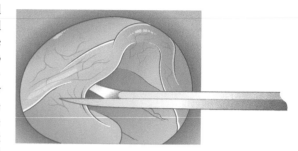

Figure 23.2 Aryepiglottoplasty. The mucosal fold between the epiglottis and the arytenoid cartilage (aryepiglottic fold) is divided.

VOCAL CORD PALSY

Vocal cord palsy can be unilateral or bilateral. It can be a difficult diagnosis, hence is often missed. The typical presentation is with respiratory distress immediately after birth, often with a weak or absent cry, feeding difficulties, aspiration and marked stridor. The degree of airway compromise depends on the position of the paralysed cord(s), and some children – especially with bilateral palsy – will require tracheostomy. Most cases resolve in time, so it is wise to persist with conservative treatment as long as the child has a safe airway. Investigations should include imaging; skilled ultrasonography can demonstrate the paretic cord. MRI can demonstrate intracranial pathology in bilateral palsy, or a mediastinal lesion compressing the recurrent laryngeal nerve in unilateral palsy. Some cases occur following cardiac surgery but more often the aetiology is unknown. Definitive treatment in the form of cord lateralisation or, in some cases, laryngotracheal reconstruction may be needed.

LARYNGEAL WEB

Webbing or atresia can occur at various sites in the larynx, but most commonly at the level of the vocal cords (**Figure 23.3**). Mild cases may not require intervention, but severe cases where there is near-complete airway obstruction will need definitive surgical repair, often involving laryngotracheal reconstruction. A preliminary tracheostomy can be life-saving. A laryngeal web may seem fairly innocuous when discovered at endoscopy, and it can be tempting to divide it in the expectation that this will give immediate and sustained relief of airway obstruction, but almost always the visible 'web' is the upper limit of a longer atretic segment, and more extensive surgery is required. Balloon dilatation is an increasingly popular strategy to expand the airway.

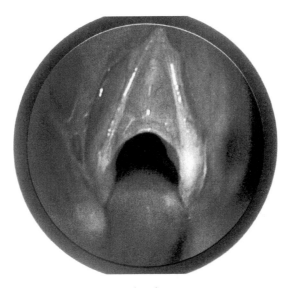

Figure 23.3 Laryngeal web.

CONGENITAL LARYNGOTRACHEAL STENOSIS

The congenital form is a type of atresia and, in severe cases, can amount to near-total agenesis of the airway, which is fatal. Milder forms, particularly isolated *subglottic stenosis (SGS)* can present with repeated episodes of stridor, especially when the child develops a respiratory infection, and can elude diagnosis for many years. The diagnosis is made at rigid endoscopy. Children with Down syndrome are particularly susceptible.

Most cases can be managed conservatively in the expectation that the calibre of the airway will expand as the child gets older. More severe cases may need laryngotracheal reconstruction or cricoid resection (see Chapter 24). '*Complete tracheal rings*' is a particularly difficult condition where the entire tracheal circumference is encircled by rigid cartilaginous rings rather than the normal horseshoe shape which does not extend to the posterior tracheal wall. This is especially challenging surgically (slide tracheoplasty) and requires very highly specialised care.

LARYNGOTRACHEAL CLEFT

This is essentially a defect in the party wall between the larynx in front and the oesophagus behind. Mild cases (type 1) extend as far as the vocal folds, whereas the most severe (type 4) extend into the trachea as far as the carina. There is a strong association with other anomalies, particularly tracheo-oesophageal fistula (TOF). Presentation may be delayed, especially in type 1 where there may be few or no symptoms. Feeding difficulties, aspiration, repeated episodes of airway obstruction and recurrent respiratory infections may alert the clinician, and the diagnosis is confirmed at endoscopy. Imaging (videofluoroscopy) can demonstrate the overspill of contrast from the oesophagus into the airway.

Type 1 cases may need no treatment or may respond to simple measures such as thickening the child's feeds. If surgery is needed, it can be performed endoscopically, freshening and apposing the mucosa in the posterior wall of the larynx. More severe cases may require tracheostomy, feeding gastrostomy, and eventual repair via laryngofissure or even open thoracotomy, with uncertain and often poor outcomes.

TRACHEO-OESOPHAGEAL FISTULA

TOF is a persistent communication between the oesophagus and the trachea, often in association with atresia of the oesophagus. There are several anatomical variants, the commonest being an atretic oesophagus with the blind stump extending into the mediastinum and a distal oesophageal remnant communicating with the trachea lower down (**Figure 23.4**). A much rarer variety, but of particular importance to the ORL specialist, is the 'H' fistula where there is no oesophageal atresia and an intact trachea but there is a fistulous communication between the two, typically in the mediastinum. The fistula opening in the trachea can be found at tracheo-bronchoscopy in a child with recurrent unexplained respiratory infections, but it can be very elusive.

TOF is often associated with other congenital abnormalities including vertebral, anal, cardiac, tracheal, renal and limb (VACTERL). Tracheomalacia is common, and some children will require tracheostomy in addition to surgical repair of the TOF, often for a prolonged period. 'Aortopexy' – anchoring the aortic arch which is closely attached to the anterior tracheal wall – to the ventral surface of the sternum may help

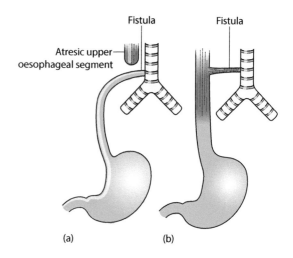

Figure 23.4 (a) Blind-ending oesophageal pouch and a fistula between the lower oesophageal lumen and the trachea. (b) 'H'-type. The fistula connects the oesophageal and tracheal lumens directly. A 'pit' may be evident on the posterior tracheal wall at tracheoscopy.

to hoist the trachea forward and increase the patency of the lumen.

HAEMANGIOMA

Haemangiomas ('birth marks') are common, mostly occurring on the skin. Not all are obvious at birth, and they proliferate during early infancy only to become apparent during the first few months. Airway haemangiomas are typically in the subglottic region, sometimes but by no means always in association with cutaneous lesions. The child presents with worsening stridor from about 2 months, eventually progressing to severe airway obstruction. Late presentation is uncommon but the child may be *in extremis* by the time they get to see an otolaryngologist. The diagnosis is made at endoscopy when a smooth, soft (pear-shaped) subglottic swelling is seen. Imaging can help to delineate it.

Even if the airway obstruction is incomplete, active treatment is needed as the lesion will grow rapidly before it involutes and may cause complete airway obstruction if untreated. Treatment in the past was surgical, often involving a tracheostomy or prolonged steroid therapy, but the method of choice now is the use of propranolol over a period of about 4–6 weeks under the supervision of a paediatrician or a cardiologist with expertise in this area. Surgery may be appropriate in some circumstances and, ideally, these children will be managed in a multidisciplinary team which includes an otolaryngologist. Most infantile hemangiomas disappear in childhood if left untreated.

VASCULAR COMPRESSION

While not abnormalities of the tracheobronchial tree, some vascular anomalies can compress the trachea and present as airway obstruction. The commonest of these is a double aortic arch (*vascular ring*). The aorta splits into two segments, one passing behind the oesophagus and one in front of the trachea, compressing both. An aberrant innominate artery may cross and compress the trachea just above the carina (*vascular sling*), and there are some less common variants. The otolaryngologist may notice an indentation in the anterior tracheal wall at endoscopy, and the diagnosis is confirmed by imaging. Early referral to the paediatric cardiac service is advised, and the prognosis is usually excellent.

TRACHEOMALACIA

Partial or complete collapse of the trachea or bronchi during respiration is caused by a lack of rigidity in the developing cartilage. To some degree, this is physiological, but it can be severe and even life-threatening. It is 'primary' if it occurs due to segmental or complete maldevelopment of the tracheal rings, and 'secondary' if it occurs as a result of compression, (e.g. by a vascular ring or in association with a TOF) where it can complicate surgical repair. In severe cases, the child will have what parents and physicians often refer to as 'dying spells' when the airway compromise gives rise to apnoea and cyanosis, especially brought about by expiration as the smaller airways close off. Diagnosis is confirmed by endoscopy, often supplemented by contrast bronchography, especially if there is a prominent element of bronchomalacia.

Treatment is difficult and may involve pressure ventilation – continuous positive airway pressure (CPAP) or bilevel positive airway pressure (BiPAP) – until there is spontaneous improvement. A tracheostomy may be needed to facilitate ventilation or to bypass a malacic segment. Some cases respond to 'aortopexy', where the aorta is hitched forward and anchored to the sternum, thus pulling the mediastinal structures, including the trachea, with it and opening the lumen.

RARE LARYNGOTRACHEOBRONCHIAL CONDITIONS

Laryngeal cysts and laryngocoeles may be congenital. A *laryngocoele* is an outpouching of the laryngeal mucosa which projects beyond the confines of the larynx; a *saccular cyst* is a discrete, fluid-filled 'sac' which does not communicate with the airway but develops in the mucosa of the airway, often in the vallecula or the glottis. If they obstruct the airway, they can be removed surgically. A bifid epiglottis, anterior laryngeal cleft and the rare *cri du chat syndrome* (a 'mewing' cry due to persistent opening of the posterior glottis during phonation in association with microcephaly, now known to be due to a partial deletion of chromosome 5) are among the findings that can be noted at laryngotracheoscopy. Congenital *bronchial cysts* and rare *mediastinal tumours* may sometimes present to the otolaryngologist.

KEY POINTS

- Laryngomalacia is common. Mild symptoms need no intervention. Consider endoscopy if symptoms are severe, the baby is failing to thrive or there is diagnostic uncertainty.
- Propranolol is the first-choice management strategy for airway haemangiomas. Surgery is now rarely needed.

FURTHER READING

Laryngomalacia. BMJ best practice guideline. Available at: https://bestpractice.bmj.com/topics/en-gb/754 (accessed 6 June 2022)

24

ACQUIRED LARYNGOTRACHEAL DISEASE

INTRODUCTION

Acute infections – including *diphtheria* and *epiglottitis* – were an important cause of childhood morbidity and mortality until well into the twentieth century and major indications for tracheostomy in children. Cicatrisation of the subglottis due to ET intubation assumed importance in the latter part of the century as neonatal care improved and paediatric intensive care facilities – with their reliance on assisted ventilation via indwelling ET tubes – developed. Laryngotracheal infections remain an important global health issue but vaccination programmes, improved knowledge and understanding of neonatal care and better ET tubes have all greatly reduced the importance of both infections and iatrogenic airway problems in the developed world.

INFECTION

■ Acute epiglottitis

Typically due to *Haemophilus influenza B* (Hib), this condition was rampant for much of the twentieth century. Widespread implementation of Hib vaccination in children has greatly reduced its incidence, but cases still occur occasionally due to vaccine failure, and rarely due to organisms other than Hib, particularly in vulnerable children such as those with compromised immune systems. Children aged between about 2 and 7 years are especially susceptible. They present with a rapidly progressing febrile illness, sore throat and painful swallow. Airway obstruction may not be immediately apparent but can very quickly progress. Settle and calm the child as much as possible and admit them to hospital for urgent observation and treatment. Avoid anything that might precipitate laryngospasm such as over-enthusiastic examination, the tongue depressor or endoscope until you are satisfied that the airway is secured, usually by ET intubation. Commence IV antibiotics and carefully monitor the airway until the swollen oedematous epiglottis and the surrounding structures have returned to normal before considering extubation. This is preferably accomplished in the controlled setting of a PICU.

DOI: 10.1201/9780429019128-24

Acute laryngotracheobronchitis

Acute laryngotracheobronchitis (ALTB) is commonly referred to as 'croup', which describes the typically harsh cough which accompanies a common viral infection in children. It is more prevalent in the winter months and can be due to one of a variety of viruses including the respiratory syncytial virus (RSV) or a parainfluenza virus. The usual age of onset is about 18 months. The mucosa of the larynx, trachea and bronchi becomes suffused and oedematous with a marked reduction in the calibre of the airway and the child becomes progressively more distressed. In severe cases stridor is marked, leading on to respiratory failure. Mild cases can be managed at home. The response to systemic steroids (oral dexamethasone 0.4 mg per kg) is usually very rapid, but more severe cases will need hospital admission for observation with serial monitoring (pulse oximetry), nebulised adrenaline, oxygen therapy and sometimes, in exceptional circumstances, airway support including ET intubation.

Some children are prone to recurrent episodes of 'croup' and may be referred to the ORL service for investigation to rule out an underlying cause. Very occasionally, cases of undiagnosed laryngotracheal stenosis present in this way and endoscopy can be reassuring, but more often there is no structural abnormality and the symptoms are due to mucosal hypersensitivity. Often, these children go on to develop bronchial asthma and continued monitoring and surveillance under the supervision of a paediatrician may be needed.

Bacterial (membranous) tracheitis

This is a much more serious condition and can complicate an apparently innocuous bout of croup. The tracheal mucosa becomes infected with sloughing and exudation due to pyogenic bacteria such as *Staphylococcus aureus*, *Streptococcus pyogenes* and *Strep. pneumonia*. The child will require admission to a PICU and is at risk of overwhelming sepsis and of potentially fatal mediastinitis. The otolaryngologist may be required to undertake a therapeutic airway endoscopy, removing exudate and slough.

Recurrent respiratory papillomatosis

RRP is a now uncommon condition occurring both in adults and children (juvenile-onset recurrent respiratory papillomatosis, JORRP) characterised by warty excrescences in the respiratory tract (**Figure 24.1**). It is caused by the *human papillomavirus (HPV)*, principally types 6 and 11, hence the expectation that it may become a very rare condition as widespread HPV vaccination programmes are established. Transmission is thought to be via the birth canal, although cases have been recorded in babies born by Caesarian section. Colonisation of the maternal genital tract – usually asymptomatic but sometimes in association with genital warts – is common (25% or more), but JORRP is very rare so it is likely that there are some host susceptibility factors at play. JORRP presents with hoarseness in children typically from the age of 4 years and upwards although it may manifest in younger children, usually an indication of more aggressive disease. Untreated, the exophytic lesions will proliferate and obstruct the airway. Diagnosis is confirmed at endoscopy by observing the characteristic warty lesions, and treatment is surgical.

The preferred technique nowadays is repeated removal of the lesions at endoscopy by a microdebrider. Of the various excision techniques – which include the use of the CO_2 laser and Coblator™ – this seems to produce

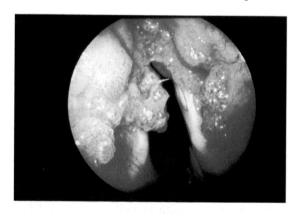

Figure 24.1 The larynx in RRP. The warty excrescences cause dysphonia progressing to airway obstruction.

the least damage to surrounding tissues. Repeated surgeries are the norm, some children requiring endoscopy only every 6 months and some needing disease debulking every few weeks to maintain a safe airway. Resolution is expected by puberty, but some children have recalcitrant disease persisting into adulthood. The lesions may progress at an alarming rate and cause concern regarding impending airway compromise, but traditional advice is to avoid tracheostomy except in the most extreme circumstances. Seeding of disease within the trachea and bronchi can be fatal, causing lung cavitation and respiratory failure, and there is a small risk of malignant transformation.

Medical treatments are available as an adjunct to surgery, but the evidence for their use is uncertain.

Interferon, acyclovir, ribavirin and various vaccines have been tried. There is some evidence to support the therapeutic use of the HPV vaccine. Cidofovir (an antiviral agent originally developed to treat CMV) has enjoyed a vogue as an intralesional agent injected at the time of surgery and, while there have been good reports of efficacy, there is uncertainty with regard to the potential long-term toxicity.

Vaccination of adolescent girls and, in many countries, boys as well has begun to reduce the prevalence of genital HPV, with an expected reduction in the incidence of both JORRP and carcinoma of the uterine cervix in women already apparent in many countries.

INTUBATION TRAUMA AND EXTUBATION FAILURE

Premature babies, often with multiple significant and life-threatening medical issues, are now routinely managed on highly specialised neonatal and paediatric intensive care units (PICUs) with excellent survival prospects. Many require assisted ventilation, typically with the help of an indwelling ET tube, sometimes for long periods. As this practice became commonplace from the 1960s onwards, it became apparent that a number of children developed scarring and stenosis of the airway, presumably as a direct consequence of prolonged or traumatic intubation. Trauma at the level of the cords caused glottic webs; trauma further down caused SGS. Tracheostomy was the inevitable consequence until surgical techniques to reconstruct the airway became widely available.

Severe SGS is less common nowadays, but iatrogenic injury to the larynx and trachea still occurs. Granulation tissue on the free edge of the cords is a not uncommon finding at endoscopy. Mucosal cysts in the larynx and upper trachea are now frequently identified in intubated babies and may compromise extubation. Large fluid-filled cysts may require uncapping at endoscopy (**Figure 24.2**). Failure to extubate a baby due to swelling of the subglottic mucosa may respond to systemic steroids for a few days, followed by another attempt at extubation under endoscopic vision to check for cysts, swelling and oedema. Balloon dilatation

under endoscopic control has become more widely available and may be helpful in mild cases. The 'cricoid split', using a vertical incision through the midline of the cricoid cartilage, often possible by an endoscopic approach, may permit the introduction of a slightly larger ET tube for a few days to enable another attempt at extubation, but repeated failure suggests that SGS has occurred and more radical intervention is needed, sometimes necessitating a temporary tracheostomy.

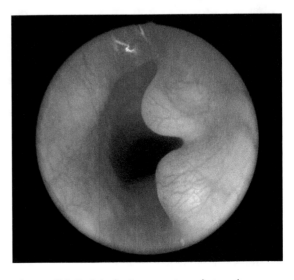

Figure 24.2 Subglottic cysts viewed at endoscopy.

SGS implies irreversible scarring of the subglottic airway (**Figure 24.3**). It is traditionally graded by the Cotton–Meyer classification depending on the extent to which the calibre (cross-sectional area) of the airway is reduced (**Box 24.1**).

Grade 1 and some grade 2 cases may not require corrective surgery; steroid therapy sometimes with repeated balloon dilatation may suffice. More severe disease will need definitive correction.

Surgery for SGS is now best carried out in a limited number of centres where the child can be looked after by an experienced team. The most widely performed traditional surgery is *laryngotracheal reconstruction*

(*LTR*), using a graft, often autologous rib cartilage, to expand the scarred airway (**Figure 24.4**). Some children may be suitable for *cricotracheal resection (CTR)* with removal of the lower rim of the cricoid cartilage and part of the upper trachea and anastomosis of the free ends (**Figure 24.5**). The aim is to enable the child to manage without a tracheostomy.

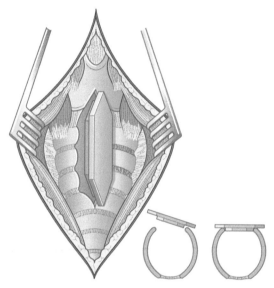

Figure 24.4 Laryngotracheal reconstruction. A linear incision is made through the midline of the larynx (laryngofissure) and extended into the upper trachea. A rib graft is fashioned and inserted in the resultant defect to expand the stenosed airway.

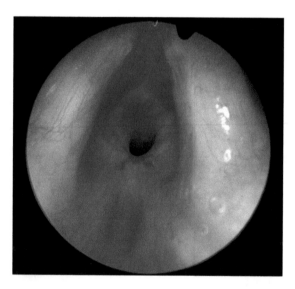

Figure 24.3 Subglottic stenosis – endoscopic appearance.

Box 24.1 Cotton–Meyer classification of SGS

- Grade 1: <50% reduction
- Grade 2: 50–70% reduction
- Grade 3: >70–90% reduction
- Grade 4: 100% occlusion

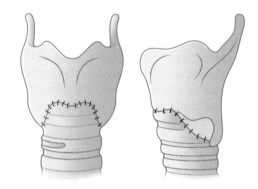

Figure 24.5 Cricotracheal resection. Cartilage is resected and the resultant free edges anastomosed as shown.

LARYNGOTRACHEAL TRAUMA

Not all cases of laryngeal trauma are iatrogenic. Swallowed caustic substances can cause serious and life-changing injuries to the airway, and blunt trauma, although uncommon, is occasionally reported as is thermal injury due to inhalation of hot air during exposure to fires.

VOICE DISORDERS

Vocal cord nodules in children may cause hoarseness and are best managed conservatively, ideally with the help of a speech and language therapist (SALT). Cysts, polyps and very rarely neoplasms may occur in the larynx and present with dysphonia. Vocal cord palsy may be iatrogenic following thoracotomy with injury to the recurrent laryngeal nerve. It is usually temporary, but long-standing cases may respond to injection techniques.

FURTHER READING

Meites E, Stone L, Amiling R et al. Significant declines in juvenile-onset recurrent respiratory papillomatosis following human papillomavirus (HPV) vaccine introduction in the United States. *Clin Infect Dis.* 2021;73(5):885–90. doi: 10.1093/cid/ciab171.

KEY POINTS

- Acute epiglottitis is an acute airway emergency. Admit the child, avoid any instrumentation of the airway (including the tongue depressor) and start antibiotics immediately.
- The management of 'croup' has been greatly improved by widespread use of steroids (dexamethasone).
- RRP is a viral disease. HPV vaccination should make this already rare condition even less common.
- Think of RRP in any child with unexplained hoarseness. Make sure you get a view of the larynx.
- Avoid surgery for children with vocal cord nodules if at all possible. Refer to a SALT.

25
TRACHEOSTOMY

INTRODUCTION

Tracheotomy refers to a surgical opening in the trachea. It is used to bypass the upper (pharyngeal and laryngeal) airway and to permit air entry into the trachea and bronchi. When the opening has formed a mature track from the tracheal lumen to the skin of the neck (i.e. it includes a 'stoma'), this is a *tracheostomy*, but the terms are used interchangeably. Tracheotomy in children may be lifesaving.

INDICATIONS

Multiple medical and surgical conditions in children lead the clinician to consider tracheostomy but remember that this is just one of a number of options that may be appropriate for dealing with an obstructed airway. Techniques for providing airway support and maintenance in children have improved (**Box 25.1**). The three main categories of indications for tracheostomy are to *bypass obstruction*, to *facilitate ventilation* and to permit *tracheal aspiration*.

> **Box 25.1 Avoiding tracheostomy: some techniques for airway support**
>
> - High-flow oxygen via a facemask
> - Nebulised adrenaline 2 mL (1 in 1000)
> - Steroids – dexamethasone 0.4 mg per kg can be given orally
> - A Guedel airway
> - Nasopharyngeal airway (NPA)
> - Endotracheal (ET) intubation
> - Non-invasive ventilation, e.g. via nasal prongs or a face mask

TECHNIQUE

Fortunately, emergency tracheotomy is very rarely indicated. If you cannot gain access to a child's airway in any other way – for example, if the larynx is completely obstructed and the child is unable to breathe – then you may need to make an emergency opening into the larynx via the cricothyroid membrane. A wide-bore needle

DOI: 10.1201/9780429019128-25

is best; definitive measures can be considered once the immediate crisis is resolved. This is only really feasible in the older child, as the cricothyroid membrane is not well developed before the age of about 3 years.

As with any surgical intervention, detailed preoperative counselling of the parent(s) and fully informed consent are vital. Formal tracheotomy is usually undertaken in controlled conditions in a fully anaesthetised child with an ET tube in place (**Figure 25. 1**).

The author's preference is for a transverse incision, securing haemostasis with bipolar diathermy. Remove a pad of subcutaneous fat (**Figure 25.2**) and continue the dissection staying in the midline, down to the pretracheal fascia. The isthmus of the thyroid gland may be in the way and can be divided, but it is often easy simply to displace it. When the fascia is cleared from the tracheal cartilage, you should be able to see the rings clearly. Be certain you have identified the rings; check with your assistant and feel the ET tube by rolling it gently between finger and thumb before placing two 'stay sutures' just lateral to the midline, one on either side (**Box 25.2**). You can then use these to help open the tracheotomy and to facilitate insertion of a tracheostomy tube (**Figure 25.3**).

Liaise closely with the anaesthetist throughout, and make sure the tube is the right length. If it is too short, it will pop out of the neck; if it is too long, it will go into the bronchus on one side and the other lung will not be ventilated. Take care that the tube is the right calibre and length. The size of the ET tube is a good guide. Some important differences between adult and paediatric tracheostomy are shown in **Box 25.3**.

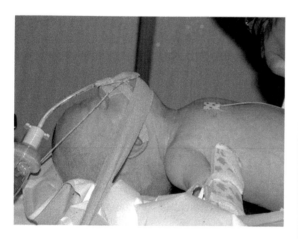

Figure 25.1 Child positioned for tracheostomy.

> ### Box 25.2 Tracheostomy
>
> - Keep your dissection to the midline.
> - Find the tracheal rings and do not make an incision in the tracheal wall until you are certain you have identified them.
> - Liaise closely with the anaesthetist to make sure the airway is safe before you insert a tracheotomy tube.

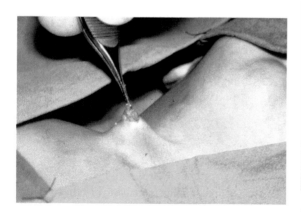

Figure 25.2 Removal of a fat pad.

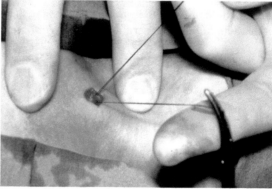

Figure 25.3 Stay sutures facilitate safe positioning of the tube.

COMPLICATIONS

These may be immediate (perioperative), delayed (i.e. in the days post-surgery) or late. Some important complications are shown in **Box 25.4**.

POSTOPERATIVE CARE

Postoperative care starts in the operating room. Check the tube well before you open the trachea and have a range of sizes ready. Secure the tube well so it does not pop out. Make sure the tapes holding it in place are neither too loose nor too tight. You should be able to comfortably get your index finger between the child's neck and the tape. Leave the stay sutures in and tape them down (**Figure 25.4**). Carers looking after the child need to know what to do in the event of an emergency. Have a spare tube with an introducer at the bedside at all times and ensure adequate suction and humidification facilities are available.

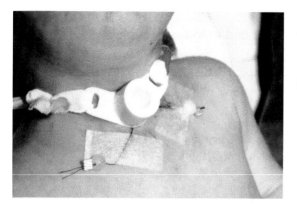

The child needs constant nursing care and observation for the first 24 hours, with easy access to a skilled resuscitation team. The tube can be changed after about 5 days, by which time the tract will be mature and stable.

Figure 25.4 Tracheostomy tube in position.

TRACHEOSTOMY TUBES IN CHILDREN

Tubes have improved greatly in recent years. Silastic tubes are flexible yet strong, cause less tissue reaction than older rubber tubes, and are easily inserted by parents and carers provided they are well trained. Children's tubes typically have no inner tube due to the narrow calibre of the airway, and fenestrated tubes are very rarely used due to the risk of excessive granulation tissue. Cuffed tubes may be needed to help ventilation but, in general, are best avoided for long-term use.

HOME CARE

Many tracheotomised children are managed at home. This can be a daunting prospect for parents, carers and teachers, all of whom need support and training. Parents need to understand that a tracheotomy, although often lifesaving, has a series of adverse effects and comes with some risk. A child with a tracheostomy will need regular suctioning of the chest to remove secretions. In the early stages, the child will be unable to speak as they will not be able to project air into the larynx. This will affect the child's ability to cry, which many parents find very distressing. Inspired air needs to be moistened and ideally warmed, as the nose and upper airway are bypassed. A period of several weeks' inpatient care is usually required to train parents about suction, tube change technique, humidification, stoma care and resuscitation. Looking after a child with a tracheostomy will have a profound effect on the family dynamics, work patterns, etc., and can be highly demanding. Good community support with access to skilled nurses and regular follow-up makes for a far smoother path for parent and child.

DECANNULATION

Sometimes, a child is best managed with a tracheotomy indefinitely but, in most cases, decannulation (removal of the tracheostomy tube) can be planned once the condition that required the tracheostomy has resolved. There are different protocols and planning regimes but, generally, a few days' inpatient care to assess the airway and ensure the child can manage without the tracheostomy tube is needed.

TRACHEOCUTANEOUS FISTULA

A persistent leakage of mucus and air through the stoma is not uncommon even long after successful decannulation, especially if the tube has been in place for a prolonged period (**Figure 25.5**). Often the 'fistula' will heal spontaneously but, if it persists for more than about 6 months, it may need surgical closure.

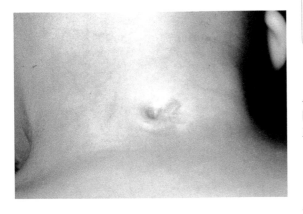

Figure 25.5 Tracheocutaneous fistula.

FURTHER READING

Manchester University NHS Foundation Trust. National tracheostomy safety project. Available at: https://www.tracheostomy.org.uk/healthcare-staff/emergency-care-child (accessed 14 January 2022).

26

CONGENITAL DISORDERS OF THE NECK

INTRODUCTION

The development of the head and neck in the embryo is complex, and it is no surprise that congenital anomalies in this region are fairly commonplace. Disorders in infants and children that present with a neck mass are very different from those that occur in adults and require a different approach to investigation and management. Congenital disorders include developmental cysts, vascular anomalies and abnormalities of the embryonic pharyngeal arches. Not all of these are immediately apparent at birth; they may present when the child is a little older.

DERMOID CYST

The lines of fusion during embryonic development may close with the inclusion of epithelial cells. These cells may be of ectodermal and mesodermal origin, with sebaceous glands and sometimes hair follicles. The cells produce a cheesy, sebaceous material and gradually enlarge to present as a cyst. The typical position is in the midline of the neck where it may be confused with the more common thyroglossal duct cyst. Clinically, a dermoid cyst forms into a firm mobile mass, which, because it is not attached to the tongue base, does not protrude on swallowing. Imaging is the first-line investigation. An ultrasound scan will show a discrete cyst, with – in contrast with a thyroglossal cyst – no 'track' extending upwards (**Figure 26.1**).

Treatment is surgical, for aesthetic reasons but not least to confirm the diagnosis. A simple cystectomy is adequate but, as the distinction between a dermoid and a thyroglossal cyst is not always made preoperatively, many children will have the more extensive 'Sistrunk's' procedure. Dermoid cysts can present in other sites, notably the dorsum of the nose (see Chapter 17).

DOI: 10.1201/9780429019128-26

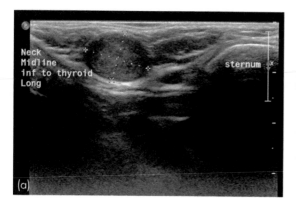
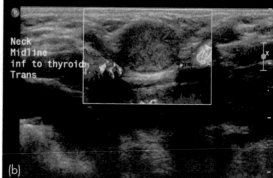

Figure 26.1 Dermoid cyst: (a) longitudinal view, (b) transverse view.

THYROGLOSSAL DUCT CYST

The thyroid gland develops high in the neck at the tongue base and descends behind the hyoid during intrauterine life to take up its position encircling the trachea and the alae of the thyroid cartilage. Descent is via a lumened structure – the 'thyroglossal duct' – which eventually atrophies. If the duct persists, it may form a cyst, typically in the midline but sometimes a little to one side. Clinically, this is evident as a firm swelling, said to move on protrusion of the tongue due to its attachment to the tongue base. This sign is inconstant and unreliable. The swelling is not always in contact with the tongue, and the diagnosis should be confirmed by imaging. Ultrasound scanning will show a cyst, and the radiologist may be able to demonstrate a tract going to the tongue base. It is prudent to ask the radiologist to note the presence of a normal thyroid, as there have been rare reports of thyroglossal cysts that contain the only remaining functioning thyroid epithelium. CT and MRI scanning are not usually needed.

Treatment is surgical. Thyroglossal cysts may become infected, making subsequent surgery more difficult due to scarring. Simple cystectomy is inadequate and liable to lead to recurrence. The 'Sistrunk's' procedure is the classical operation for a thyroglossal cyst and includes removal not only of the cyst but of the tissue above, extending to the tongue base and including the mid-portion of the hyoid bone (**Figure 26.2**). The important thing is not to leave any residual epithelial cells which could cause the cyst to reform. Wide excision to include adjacent soft tissue which could harbour cell rests or a remnant of the tract is the key to successful first-time surgery.

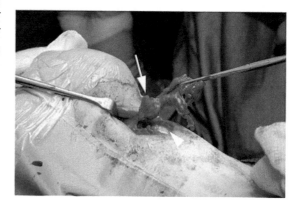

Figure 26.2 Excision of a thyroglossal duct cyst.

LINGUAL THYROID

This is a rare anomaly in which some or all of the thyroid gland fails to descend and is found at the level of the foramen caecum of the tongue. It may be the only functioning thyroid tissue. It is usually asymptomatic but may cause dysphagia, airway obstruction or bleeding. MRI scanning demonstrates the mass well.

If treatment is required, it is usually medical, i.e. suppression of activity and growth by thyroid stimulating hormone (TSH) under the supervision of an endocrinologist. Surgery is very rarely needed.

THE BRANCHIAL ARCHES

The structures of the head and neck in the developing embryo are derived from a series of bars of mesenchymal tissue – the 'branchial' or 'pharyngeal' arches. Six arches are described, and they are separated by external clefts and internal pouches. The first 'arch' gives rise to the maxilla and mandible, and the second gives rise to some of the structures that form the ear. Major anomalies (agenesis or partial agenesis) of these arches form the basis of some craniofacial anomalies such as hemifacial microsomia and mandibulofacial dysostosis. More commonly, developmental anomalies may give rise to cysts (fluid-filled sacs), sinuses (blind-ending tracts) or fistulas (abnormal communications between two structures, e.g. the skin and the pharynx), which can become infected and will often require surgery.

First-arch anomalies give rise to cysts, sinuses or fistulas in the pre-auricular area. They are highly challenging surgically because of the potentially close relationship to the facial nerve (**Figure 26.3**).

Second-arch fistulas are the commonest manifestation of arch anomalies to require surgery. They usually present in older children or in young adults, sometimes following one or more infections. The external opening is in the skin of the upper neck and the internal orifice may be deep in the pharynx, often within the tonsil. Surgical excision involves following the tract upwards to its internal opening, taking care to navigate the carotid sheath and the hypoglossal nerve.

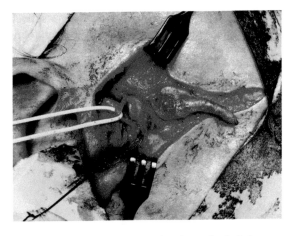

Figure 26.3 Excision of a first branchial cleft tract. The tract has been dissected out and separated from its opening in the floor of the ear canal. The yellow sloop is over the facial nerve trunk.

A third or fourth branchial cleft abnormality can give rise to recurrent neck abscess, often involving the thyroid gland, as these arches are closely related to the thyroid and parathyroid glands. The typical anomaly is a sinus extending from the pyriform fossa to deep in the neck. Surgical excision including a part of the thyroid lobe was the traditional approach, but some surgeons now advocate endoscopy with identification of the pharyngeal orifice which can be cauterised.

VASCULAR AND LYMPHATIC MASSES

These are now classified as either 'vascular tumours' or 'vascular malformations'. 'Haemangiomas' or 'birth marks' are the commonest variety of vascular tumour, and are usually innocuous, self-limiting and require no treatment. They may cause alarming swelling, for example in the parotid gland where they can be mistaken for a malignant tumour (see Chapter 28). Biopsy is not often needed as the radiological features (particularly MRI scanning) are so distinctive. If they encroach on important structures – notably the orbit or the airway – they may need to be more actively treated. In recent years, propranolol has been found to limit growth, and steroids, both systemic and intralesional, are sometimes used. Laser therapy or, in very rare cases, surgical excision may be required.

The commonest 'vascular malformation' in paediatric practice is a lymphangioma. This is a cystic mass, sometimes unilocular (macrocystic) but more often multilocular (microcystic), which results from abnormal development of the lymphatic system. They can be extremely large and may be made up of complex interdigitating processes that extend throughout the head and neck and are almost impossible to safely remove surgically. They may cause functional problems (e.g. airway obstruction and dysphagia) and are a source of major concern because of their aesthetic appearance. The diagnosis is clinical, confirmed by imaging; MRI scanning is especially helpful (**Figure 26.4**).

Treatment may be expectant in small lesions, but sclerotherapy using a variety of sclerosant materials (e.g. OK-432, an inactive strain of *Strep. pyogenes*) under the supervision of an interventional radiologist has become popular in recent years.

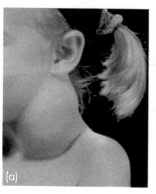 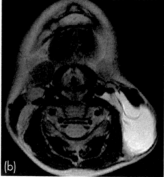 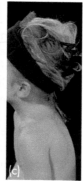

Figure 26.4 (a–c) Large lymphangioma.

FIBROMATOSIS COLLI

Previously known as 'sternomastoid tumour', this condition is characterised by torticollis and a lump in the sternomastoid muscle. The aetiology is unknown but it is most likely an idiopathic intense fibrosis of the muscle tissue. It presents in the newborn. Early recognition and intensive treatment with physiotherapy are essential to reduce the risk of permanent deformity of the neck.

Advances in prenatal imaging are now such that some congenital masses are diagnosed *in utero* (**Figure 26.5**). This means that the obstetrician/neonatologist can plan for immediate intervention in the event of a life-threatening lesion of the head and neck, such as a lesion that might cause immediate airway compromise (congenital high airway obstruction syndrome, CHAOS). An immediate tracheotomy or ET intubation while the newborn baby is still receiving placental support is termed *ex utero* intrapartum treatment (EXIT).

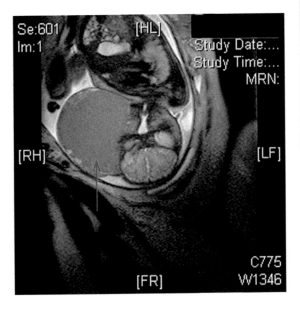

Figure 26.5 Scan of expectant mother showing baby with large extracranial mass.

KEY POINTS

- A simple 'cystectomy' is inadequate for a thyroglossal duct cyst and risks recurrence. Remove a good cuff of tissue around the cyst to include a portion of the hyoid bone and follow the track upwards to the tongue base.
- Imaging is the first-line investigation for almost all neck masses. An ultrasound scan under the supervision of an experienced paediatric radiologist is often all that is needed.
- Surgery for cysts, fistulas and sinuses to the branchial arches is demanding, with a risk to the cranial nerves. Refer to an experienced surgeon and consider facial nerve monitoring.

FURTHER READING

Trimble KG, McCadden L. Cysts and sinuses of the head and neck. In Watkinson JC, Clarke RW, Aldren CP et al (eds). *Scott-Brown's Otolaryngology, Head and Neck Surgery*, 8th edn. CRC Press; 2018.

27

ACQUIRED DISORDERS OF THE NECK

INTRODUCTION

Masses can arise from any of the structures in the neck including lymph nodes, the thyroid gland and the salivary glands. Enlargement may be in response to physiological stimuli but can be due to pathology, causing parental alarm and needing investigation and management. Lymph node enlargement – usually benign and of no pathological significance – is by far the commonest cause of a neck mass in children.

CERVICAL LYMPHADENOPATHY

The lymph nodes in the neck enlarge in response to infections, mainly viral, in the upper respiratory tract. Fluctuation in size of these nodes is therefore physiological, and part of the process whereby the child develops immunity to common upper respiratory pathogens. *Lymphadenopathy* is probably a misnomer, given the ubiquitous nature of cervical lymph node enlargement in children. A finding of one or more enlarged neck nodes in a child is a frequent cause of referral to the ORL service and may cause a great deal of parental distress. The parent and the referring clinician will be anxious to exclude malignancy, including one of the lymphoproliferative disorders.

Management starts with a careful history and examination. Multiple discrete nodes and nodes that fluctuate in size rather than continue to expand are clearly less of a worry. Small mobile nodes (up to 2 cm in diameter), long-standing nodes and bilateral symmetrical nodes are of less concern than single, large or matted nodes or nodes which have enlarged rapidly. Associated skin changes (e.g. discoloration or discharge) warrant more careful investigation. Red flags for cervical lymphadenopathy are listed in **Box 27.1**.

> **Box 27.1 Red flags for cervical lymphadenopathy**
>
> - Solitary node
> - Large node (more than 2 cm)
> - Nodes in unexpected site, e.g. supraclavicular
> - Marked asymmetry
> - 'Rubbery' or hard on palpation
> - Puckering or tethering of skin
> - Broken skin
> - Unusual ultrasound findings
> - Systemic symptoms, e.g. unexplained fever or malaise

DOI: 10.1201/9780429019128-27

The investigation of first choice is ultrasound scanning. An experienced radiologist is invaluable here and they will look for features of normal architecture in the nodes. If the hilar architecture is normal, particularly if there are adjacent nodes with a similar appearance, then the node is almost certainly a benign 'reactive' node and, provided there is nothing in the history or examination to warrant further investigation, the parents can be reassured that no intervention is needed (**Figure 27.1**). Cystic inclusions, loss of definition of the hilar 'strands' and calcification all suggest an abnormal node and will warrant further investigation, in some cases biopsy (**Figure 27.2**). Blood tests for serology to demonstrate

cytomegalovirus (CMV) or *Epstein Barr Virus* (EBV) may be useful. Infectious mononucleosis (EBV infection) is a common cause of often massive cervical adenopathy in adolescence. Diagnosis is confirmed by analysis of the blood film, which will show the atypical lymphocytes, with positive serology (monospot and Paul Bunnel tests).

If a lymphoma is suspected, the child will need a full work-up to include a chest X-ray looking at the mediastinum, blood tests and bone marrow biopsy.

Some other specific infectious agents that can cause true lymphadenopathy are *human immunodeficiency*

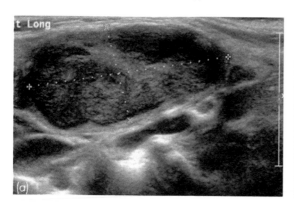 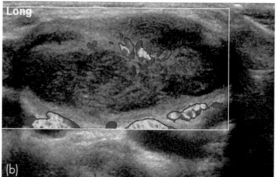

Figure 27.1 (a,b) Reactive lymph node. Ultrasound scan shows normal hilar architecture.

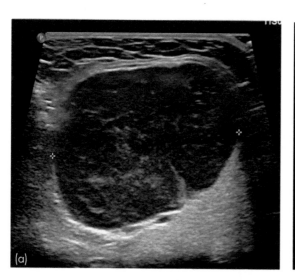 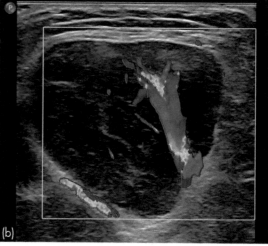

Figure 27.2 (a,b) Ultrasound scan of an abnormal node. Loss of definition of hilum.

virus (HIV), *Mycobacterium tuberculosis*, *Bartonella henselae* (cat-scratch disease), and *non-tuberculous mycobacteria* (NTM).

HIV infection in children is often associated with cervical lymphadenopathy, which may precede the development of full-blown acquired immunodeficiency syndrome (AIDS). Multiple intrasalivary gland cysts with enlargement of the parotids is another feature of cervical HIV in children. Treatment is under the supervision of a paediatric infectious diseases expert but the ORL doctor may be asked to undertake a biopsy, not least to exclude a malignancy as these children are at greatly increased risk of lymphomatous change in the neck nodes.

Cervical tuberculosis is now far less common than NTM in western communities, but it still occurs and clinicians need to be alert to make the diagnosis. It is most often found in children and adolescents who have a history of recent foreign travel and may present as a solitary 'rubbery' neck node with or without systemic symptoms and with or without discharge through the skin. Imaging may show a mass of nodes that have ruptured through the cervical fascia to form a 'dumb-bell' shaped structure, one part superficial to the fascia and one part deep ('collar-stud abscess'). Imaging may show calcification which is highly suggestive of the diagnosis. Treatment is by antituberculous chemotherapy under the supervision of an infectious diseases clinician.

NON-TUBERCULOUS MYCOBACTERIA

NTM is a chronic granulomatous infection caused by mycobacteria other than the tuberculosis bacillus, hence the earlier term *atypical mycobacteria* (*ATM*). It is becoming increasingly common and typically affects the cervical lymph nodes with a particular affinity for the intrasalivary lymphoid tissue, hence the frequency of infection in and around the parotid and submandibular regions. The age of onset is about 2–4 years, and infection is thought to occur by oral ingestion. The pathogens are soil saprophytes such as *Mycobacterium bovis*, *M. avium intracellulare* and *M. scrofulaeum*. These probably find their way into domestic water supplies and may accumulate in the limescale deposits on bathroom and shower fittings. Older children and adults seem to have developed immunity and are only at risk if they have immune dysfunction.

The lesions are slow-growing, sometimes with a characteristic violet appearance of the overlying skin (**Figure 27.3**) and sometimes with a discharging sinus that leaks a sticky effluent onto the skin. They are self-limiting and resolve over a period of months or sometimes years, but the aesthetic effects can be very distressing in the meantime. Diagnosis is largely clinical but supported by imaging, which will often show a 'collar-stud' type abscess (**Figure 27.4**) or a multicystic appearance with fluid levels

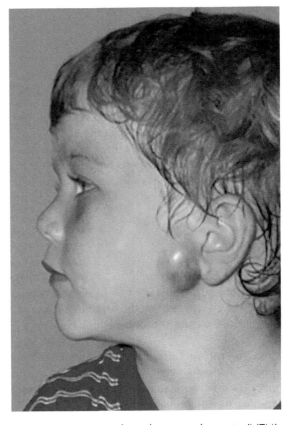

Figure 27.3 Non-tuberculous mycobacteria (NTM). Note the skin changes.

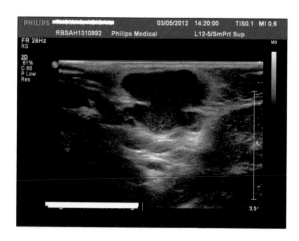

Figure 27.4 Collar-stud abscess.

within a mass of nodes. Identification of the organism by either by staining or culture is notoriously difficult. Histology, if needed, will show granulomatous inflammation but without the caseation (necrotic foci) typical of tuberculosis.

Treatment is controversial. The disease is benign and self-limiting, and the child will recover completely even if just managed by serial observation. This may leave an unsightly scar, but healing can be remarkably good and scarring is often not nearly as bad as parents fear. There is some evidence to support the use of antituberculous chemotherapy to hasten resolution, but these drugs are not without side effects and the therapeutic benefit seems to be small.

Surgery is curative if the whole of the diseased mass is removed but, as the nodes are often intimately related to the parotid and submandibular glands, there is a risk to the facial nerve trunk and to the marginal mandibular branch of the facial nerve. For this reason, many surgeons will adopt a 'wait and see' approach and only operate on easily accessible nodes or where there is repeated infection, skin changes and serious concern regarding the aesthetic outcome. The decision is clinical and made in consultation with the parents.

LYMPHOMA

Malignant tumours of the lymphoid system (the commonest malignancy in the neck in children) present with enlarged lymph nodes. Previous exposure to EBV is thought to predispose, but EBV exposure is very common and lymphomas are very uncommon. Lymphadenopathy, especially if large, prolonged or in association with fever, weight loss and systemic symptoms, may warrant urgent excision biopsy. Aspiration biopsy cytology (ABC) or fine-needle aspiration (FNA) is far less helpful in the diagnosis of neck masses in children than it is in adults and precise diagnosis and staging of lymphomas requires a good-sized specimen so the pathologist can study the detailed architecture of the lymph node.

Reed–Sternberg cells, large multinucleated and highly distinctive cells found within the affected nodes, are pathognomonic of Hodgkin's lymphoma, the most common of the lymphomas that present in children. It is more common in adolescence, and presentation before the age of 5 years is very rare.

Although a diagnosis of a lymphoma is a devastating event in the life of the child and the parents, the long-term prognosis – depending on stage, histology and treatment – may be excellent with greater than 90% survival for patients with many forms of early disease.

Lymphomas were classified as *Hodgkin's lymphoma* or *non-Hodgkin's lymphoma* based on the histology; however, as chemotherapy regimens have improved, this is now too simplistic to enable optimum therapeutic strategies. Classification and staging systems have become both more focused and more complex in recent years. Most paediatric oncologists use the World Health Organization/Revised European American Lymphoma (WHO/REAL) system to classify the histological type and the most recent modification of the Ann Arbor system to denote the stage.

The role of the ORL specialist is largely to be alert to the possibility of a lymphoma in a child with a neck mass and to undertake urgent excision biopsy when needed. Liaise with the oncology and pathology team who may require a mixture of fresh tissue and tissue sent in formalin. The child needs to be referred to a dedicated MDT and the work-up will include imaging, blood tests and possible bone marrow biopsy or harvesting.

Chemotherapy strategies are becoming increasingly more refined and tailored to the individual child, hence the importance of precise histological classification and accurate staging.

NON-INFECTIVE INFLAMMATORY CONDITIONS

A number of conditions that mimic lymphoma can give rise to enlarged neck nodes in children. *Rosai–Dorfman disease* (sinus histiocytosis with massive lymphadenopathy) presents with greatly enlarged cervical lymph nodes, fever and malaise. It is of unknown aetiology and generally self-limiting. Diagnosis is histological.

Castleman's disease is a B-cell lymphoproliferative disorder, sometimes associated with HIV infection. The diagnosis is histological. *Kikuchi–Fujimoto disease* is another histological diagnosis that can mimic lymphoma, but it is benign and self-limiting. These conditions may have an as yet unconfirmed viral aetiology.

Kawasaki syndrome – an acute multisystem vasculitis with associated cervical lymphadenopathy – has been of particular interest of late as a very similar condition is now known to be caused by COVID-19 (see Chapter 29).

Langerhans cell histiocytosis (*LCH*) occurs mainly in young children (under the age of 5 years). It is a multisystem disease, again of unknown aetiology, associated with unexplained fever, malaise and weight loss. LCH, known in the past as *Letterer–Siwe disease* or *eosinphilic granulomatosis*, is characterised by the presence of lesions – including in the cervical nodes – which have a distinctive histological appearance and may initially be mistaken for lymphoma. It can run a very aggressive course with a significant mortality (10%). Children need careful work-up and should be referred to a paediatric oncologist as some will be considered for chemotherapy.

These conditions are sometimes referred to as *pseudolymphomas* but they are not true malignancies.

NON-LYMPHOMATOUS MALIGNANCY

In western healthcare settings, cancer is second only to trauma as a cause of death in children. Around 12% of childhood cancers occur in the head and neck, the commonest being lymphoma. Neural tumours, thyroid malignancy and sarcomas (rhabdomyosarcoma) are all described and may present as a neck mass. The role of the ORL doctor is to be aware and to undertake biopsy when needed. Management is under the supervision of an oncology MDT, and survival rates for most childhood cancers have increased greatly in recent years.

Neural tumours include neuroblastoma and benign neurofibromas as well as some very aggressive neuro-ectodermal tumours.

The commonest cause of thyroid dysfunction in children worldwide is still iodine deficiency, but thyroid swellings (goitres) are often found especially in teenagers, more often in girls. They may be completely benign and associated with the hormonal changes of adolescence, needing no intervention, or they may be active nodules (e.g. follicular adenomas with associated hyperthyroidism), but the child will need investigation and work-up under the supervision of an endocrinologist. Differentiated papillary cancers, mixed papillary/follicular and rarely pure follicular cancers are not common but any thyroid mass needs careful investigation. Antecedent radiation of the head and neck is a risk factor for thyroid cancer.

Investigation starts with an ultrasound scan and, in many centres, an FNA. This is one of the few situations in children where FNA is helpful. Treatment is controversial and, as these tumours tend to be slow-growing and with very high survival rates, limited surgery is often appropriate.

The support of an MDT including an oncologist and endocrinologist is invaluable.

▐ Trauma

Injuries to the neck in children are uncommon, but we live in violent times and stab and gunshot injuries in teenagers are now frequently seen in trauma centres. Self-harm is increasingly reported in children.

Penetrating injuries that breach the platysma have the potential to involve vessels, the airway, the pharynx and oesophagus and the cervical nerves. Bleeding can be catastrophic. Initial management is in line with the general principles of resuscitation – **A**irway, **B**reathing, **C**irculation. Urgent surgical exploration may be needed especially if there are features suggestive of active bleeding or a breach of the airway, e.g. an expanding haematoma, 'bubbling' in the wound, surgical emphysema.

Blunt trauma may result from falls, sports injuries, traffic accidents and strangulation. The main concern here is airway obstruction, which can be delayed, hence the need for vigilance with admission and careful monitoring. If there is any concern that the larynx or trachea have been injured early involvement of the ORL team, to include laryngotracheoscopy – ideally under controlled conditions in the OR avoiding 'blind' **ET** intubation – is essential.

KEY POINTS

- NTM lesions improve without any treatment. Be cautious about recommending intervention, especially any surgery that could risk trauma to the facial nerve or its branches.
- Precise histopathological diagnosis of lymphoma is increasingly important as treatment regimens become more refined. Discuss with the oncologist and the pathologist before taking a biopsy and send fresh tissue straight to the laboratory. Cytology (FNA/ABC) is rarely helpful.
- A thyroid swelling warrants investigation but is usually benign.

FURTHER READING

Patel S, Burgess A. Guideline for the child presenting to hospital with lymphadenitis or a lymph node abscess. Available at: www.entuk.org/paediatric-guidelines (accessed 31 January 2022).

28 THE SALIVARY GLANDS

INTRODUCTION

Parotitis due to mumps – an extremely common childhood infection in days gone by – is now rarely seen due to widespread vaccination. Salivary masses in childhood may be caused by disease of the epithelial tissue (the parenchyma of the salivary glands) or diseases of the lymphoid tissue. Epithelial salivary tumours are rare, and disorders such as NTM (see Chapter 27), acute infections, juvenile recurrent parotitis and lymphoma are more common causes of sialomegaly. Diagnosis is often delayed. Surgery, particularly of the parotid, is especially challenging in children.

RANULA

This is a mucous retention cyst in the floor of the mouth (**Figure 28.1**). It is occasionally found in the newborn but more often presents in toddlers when it forms a smooth translucent swelling ('frog's belly'). It is thought to occur as a result of outflow obstruction in the sublingual or one of the minor salivary glands. Mucinous saliva continues to be produced, becomes encysted, and the swelling expands along the tissue planes. The cyst is found between the mucosa of the floor of the mouth and the mylohyoid muscle, usually to one side of the midline. A very large ranula will extend well into the neck (*plunging ranula*). The appearance causes parental alarm and, if very large, it can interfere with swallowing.

Diagnosis is clinical but imaging can help treatment planning. Treatment is surgical. Simple 'marsupialisation' or laying the sac open is not enough; a total cystectomy ideally with removal of adjacent salivary epithelium (i.e. the sublingual gland) is better.

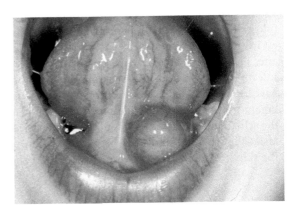

Figure 28.1 A ranula.

DOI: 10.1201/9780429019128-28

SIALADENITIS

Acute infections – particularly of the parotid – may occur due to a variety of viruses including classically the mumps virus, which causes bilateral parotitis. MMR (mumps, measles, rubella) vaccination had all but eliminated this highly contagious condition but there have been outbreaks among adolescents in particular in recent years due to poor vaccine uptake in some communities. Complications include meningitis, orchitis in boys and unilateral sensorineural hearing loss. Diagnosis is confirmed by serology.

Acute bacterial infection of the parotid (*suppurative parotitis*, **Figure 28.2**) can cause extensive cellulitis of the head and neck with abscess formation. Premature newborn infants and children with immunosuppression, poor nutrition or dental sepsis are especially at risk. Intensive treatment with IV antibiotics is needed, and occasionally abscess drainage, taking great care not to traumatise the very superficial facial nerve.

HIV infection in the parotid can give rise to multiple microcysts, and the diagnosis should be considered in unexplained parotidomegaly.

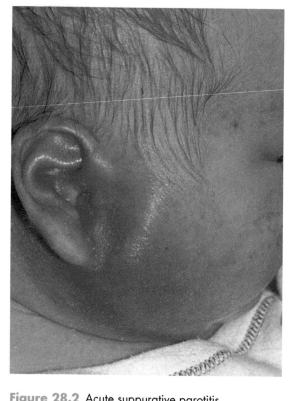

Figure 28.2 Acute suppurative parotitis.

RECURRENT PAROTITIS

This is characterised by repeated episodes of painful swelling of one or both parotids. It is commonest in older children and teenagers, and often settles after puberty. The aetiology is unknown, and both infective agents (e.g. EBV) and autoimmune factors have been implicated. Superinfection with pyogenic organisms can occur with widespread destruction of the acinar and ductal structures of the gland (sialectasia, **Figure 28.3**) and even fistula formation to the skin but, more usually, symptoms are mild and easily managed with analgesics and antibiotics as appropriate.

Contrast studies – cannulating the parotid duct and demonstrating the ductal architecture – may show strictures and ectatic ducts and may even be therapeutic in flushing debris from the gland. As with management of calculi, there is growing interest in techniques to introduce increasingly sophisticated endoscopes to the parotid duct and undertake sialendoscopic treatment.

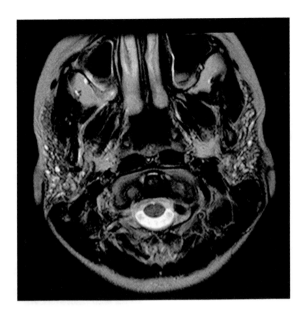

Figure 28.3 MRI scan showing extensive bilateral parotid duct ectasia.

CALCULI

Salivary stones are much more common in adults than in children. They present with painful enlargement usually of the submandibular gland. The stone is sometimes palpable in the floor of the mouth, but plain X-ray usually demonstrates it well. A course of antibiotics may be needed if the gland is infected, and it may be possible to remove the stone by massaging it toward the orifice of the duct or by opening or probing the duct orifice at surgery. There is increasing interest in and enthusiasm for sialendoscopy.

SALIVARY TUMOURS

Haemangioma of the parotid is a congenital tumour but it will not usually be apparent until the child is at least a few months old. It may grow rapidly, causing discoloration and necrosis of the skin, giving rise to extreme alarm as parents and doctors suspect an aggressive malignancy. Early referral and investigation by MRI scanning allow a definitive diagnosis, without the need for biopsy (**Figure 28.4**). The prognosis is excellent, with the natural history following the expected haemangioma pattern of a proliferative phase followed by gradual involution.

Treatment, if needed, has been greatly improved by the use of propranolol (see Chapter 28) and sometimes laser therapy. Surgery should be avoided, but very large or aggressive lesions may respond to cytotoxic agents under the supervision of a paediatric oncologist.

Lymphomas are considered in Chapter 27.

Salivary epithelial neoplasms in children are rare, but a higher proportion of childhood parotid tumours are malignant than is the case in adults, hence the need for early investigation and continued vigilance. Pleomorphic salivary adenoma (PSA) is the commonest childhood epithelial neoplasm and occurs most often in the parotid.

Malignant tumours include mucoepidermoid carcinoma and acinic cell tumours. Diagnosis is often delayed. Management may involve surgery and chemotherapy and should be undertaken by an experienced team to include a paediatric oncologist.

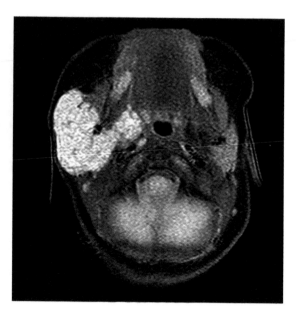

Figure 28.4 MRI scan of a parotid haemangioma.

PAROTIDECTOMY IN CHILDREN

Conditions such as branchial fistula and lymphangiomas of the head and neck may involve the parotid, and parotidectomy or a parotidectomy-type approach is often part of the surgery needed for these disorders. Parotidectomy may be part of the strategy for the treatment of malignant disease. This is highly specialised surgery and should only be undertaken by appropriately trained and experienced surgeons. Facial nerve monitoring is strongly advised. The risk to the nerve is very real, given its more superficial position in children and the frequent presence of scar tissue due to recurrent infections (e.g. in branchial fistulas). A facial paresis is a devastating complication in a child.

SIALORRHEA

'Drooling' or 'dribbling' are the colloquial terms to describe salivary overspill from the oral cavity onto the lips and the skin of the lower face. This is not true sialorrhea as salivary volume is usually normal; the issue is poor retention of saliva usually due to neurological disease which interferes with the normal swallow, i.e. neuromuscular incoordination. Some degree of 'drooling' is normal and physiological up to the age of about 4 years, but beyond this it can be very troublesome in children with neurodisability due to a variety of aetiologies, typically cerebral palsy.

Treatment at first is focused on measures to improve oromandibular posture, often with the help of a SALT and orthodontist. Pharmacological interventions include the use of antimuscarinic agents (e.g. hyoscine), frequently administered by dermal patches. ORL clinicians are often involved as part of the MDT looking after these children and are called upon when conservative measures fail. Many ORL clinicians have developed expertise in the injection of *Botulinus* toxin (Botox A) directly into the parotid and submandibular glands. Botox acts by binding to the presynaptic receptors to block acetylcholine release from parasympathetic secretomotor nerves, thus reducing salivary flow. There is a risk of extravasation and of trauma to the facial nerve, but accurate placement of the injections with the help of ultrasound guidance has made the procedure far safer. The effect is temporary, and the procedure may need to be repeated every few months.

Transposition of the submandibular ducts so that they open into the pharynx rather than via their normal distal orifices in the floor of the mouth is a now well-established technique. Many surgeons will excise the sublingual glands at the same time.

Excision of the submandibular glands is an extreme measure and only considered if all earlier approaches fail, but it is an effective way to reduce salivary flow, albeit with serious adverse effects including dental caries.

Duct ligation has been advocated in the past, but pain, swelling and recanalisation make for a difficult postoperative course and the technique is not often recommended.

KEY POINTS

- Complete removal of a ranula will give a better long-term outcome than 'marsupialisation'.
- A parotid tumour in a child is often malignant.
- Parotid surgery in children is challenging. Refer to an experienced surgeon and monitor the facial nerve throughout.

FURTHER READING

Gleeson M. Disorders of the salivary glands in children. In: Clarke R (ed.). *Pediatric Otolaryngology: Practical Clinical Management*. Thieme; 2017.

29

COVID-19 IN CHILDREN'S ORL

INTRODUCTION

Severe acute respiratory syndrome coronavirus 2 (SARS-CoV-2) – a virus isolated in Wuhan, China, in December 2019 – is the causative organism of COVID-19 (**Figure 29.1**). This new disease spread rapidly worldwide such that the WHO declared a global pandemic in March 2020. The disease mainly affects the respiratory system and manifestations may vary from no symptoms at all to significant morbidity requiring intensive ventilatory support up to organ failure and death. Higher mortality rates were associated with gender – males faring worse – obesity, and the presence of pre-existing conditions such as diabetes. Spread is primarily by droplet transmission through the respiratory mucosa but may occur by direct contact, via the gastrointestinal (GI) tract, and via the conjunctiva. Early in the course of the pandemic it became apparent that healthcare personnel, including ORL specialists, were at particular risk. Large numbers contracted COVID-19, which led to serious illness and, in many cases, death.

Vaccines were quickly developed and were approved for use at the end of 2020 and in early 2021. A worldwide vaccination programme is underway which has

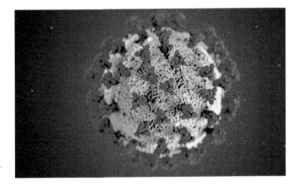

Figure 29.1 Severe acute respiratory syndrome coronavirus 2 (SARS-CoV-2), the causative organism of COVID-19.

meant greatly reduced morbidity and mortality, but COVID-19 continues to spread and intensive public health measures to reduce transmission are still in place. Widespread vaccination of adults has reduced the prevalence and severity in the adult population, but cases in children continue to rise, albeit typically with few if any symptoms and little morbidity.

ORL SERVICE DELIVERY

COVID-19 brought about seismic changes in healthcare including the provision of ORL services for adults and children. ORL interventions – particularly in children – involve very close contact

DOI: 10.1201/9780429019128-29

between clinician and child with exposure to upper respiratory secretions which form droplets containing viral particles. Healthcare workers (HCW) are particularly at risk when performing 'aerosol-generating procedures' (AGPs) such as airway endoscopy, tracheostomy, and bone-removal during tympanomastoid surgery. Examination of a child's nose or pharynx may be an AGP, particularly if the child cries or screams, and ORL staff are frequently exposed to a high viral load.

During the early stages and the peak of the pandemic, clinic visits were greatly reduced and patients with non-urgent conditions had their scheduled surgeries and outpatient consultations cancelled or rescheduled. Many consultations took place by telephone, or online via 'Zoom', 'FaceTime' or 'Teams'. Hospital visits were curtailed and children came to appointments accompanied by only one parent (**Figure 29.2**). ORL surgery was confined to urgent cases, and preoperative testing

for COVID-19 became the norm, with inevitable disruptions and delays. Staff shortages – often with little or no notice due to colleagues becoming ill or needing to isolate – made planning difficult and uncertain.

Some conditions seen in paediatric ORL declined in incidence, including acute tonsillitis, AOM and OME. The reasons are unclear but may be related to reduced exposure during 'lockdowns' and to the school closures that were implemented in many jurisdictions. Some, but not all, departments reported a 'spike' in the incidence of cases of idiopathic facial palsy in children, again for reasons that are not clear.

Many ORL interventions (e.g. tracheostomy, suction of respiratory secretions, bronchoscopy) involve the potential release of aerosols containing particles of tissue and secretions from the respiratory mucosa and are known as AGPs.

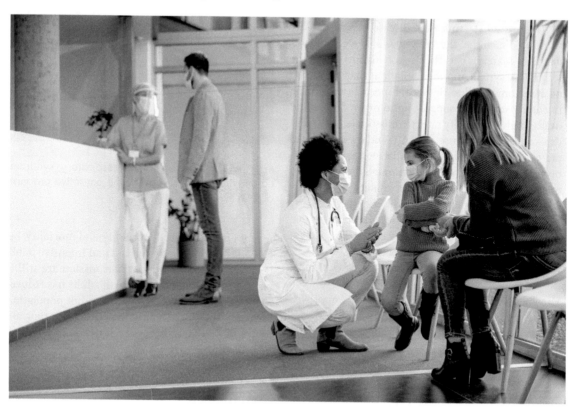

Figure 29.2 Consultations in the COVID era were very different from before. PPE, social distancing, and reduced numbers of children and parents in waiting rooms all helped to reduce environmental transmission.

Particular care and a high level of personal protective equipment (PPE) – including the use of the filtering face-piece (FFP) respirators, which offer much greater protection to the wearer than standard surgical facemasks – are needed for these interventions.

National medical associations, public health bodies and ORL societies recommended varying levels of PPE to reduce the risks of COVID-19 spread during encounters with healthcare professionals (**Figure 29.3**). Despite widespread vaccination and reduced morbidity and mortality figures, some PPE requirements are largely still in place. Hospitals and clinics introduced various changes to reduce potential exposure, including restricting the number of visitors, often permitting only one parent or carer to accompany a child on a hospital visit, keeping numbers in waiting rooms to a minimum, and mandating face coverings for parents and older children.

Testing of children, parents and healthcare personnel on a regular basis with hospital visits rescheduled in the event of a positive test made for frequent disruptions to planned operating lists and clinics. 'Telemedicine' with remote consultations by telephone or by computer links became commonplace.

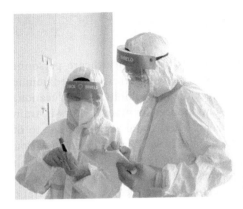

Figure 29.3 Varying levels of PPE were recommended to reduce the risks of COVID-19 spread.

Face coverings, double gloving, respirator masks, increased time intervals between consultations and longer waiting times for surgery have significantly altered the dynamics of patient and clinician interaction.

Residents and trainees inevitably had less exposure to surgical procedures, and training programmes in many cases had to be extended as a result.

Requirements are now less stringent and subject to revision, but there is no doubt that COVID-19 has brought about many changes that are here to stay. The 'new normal' looks likely to continue for some time to come.

CLINICAL FEATURES OF COVID-19 IN CHILDREN

It is now clear that children and young people (CYP) are susceptible to COVID-19 but the risk of contracting the disease is considerably lower than in adults. Symptoms tend to be minimal or absent, morbidity is much less and mortality extremely rare. Cough, fever, disturbances of taste and smell and rhinorrhoea have all been reported. The role of CYP in disease transmission is as yet unclear.

Early in the course of the pandemic, it became apparent that a small number of children infected with COVID-19 developed a serious and life-threatening illness characterised by multisystem inflammation – multisystem inflammatory syndrome in children (MIS-C). The clinical and laboratory features were not dissimilar to the findings in other multisystem inflammatory disorders in children (e.g. Kawasaki disease).

Later manifestations of COVID-19 (long COVID) are described, but the precise effects will only become known in the years to come.

Education and training of healthcare personnel was especially challenging, with a reduced number of cases for teaching, a prohibition on educational gatherings, and the need for many doctors-in-training and their teachers to take time off due to illness or the need to isolate. 'Lockdowns' in various countries involved prolonged closure of schools. The long-term effects on children's social development have yet to be determined. Parental reluctance to present for appointments, hospital policies with regard to waiting lists for routine visits, and a growing backlog of children who were not seen during the height of the pandemic have all made for difficult times ahead.

It is likely that reduced exposure to the common viral illnesses of childhood during periods of 'lockdown' or school closures will result in lowered immunity to these conditions, and many children's services are already seeing a surge in admissions of children with, for example, RSV.

The legacy of the pandemic on long-term health and well-being is yet to be determined.

FURTHER READING

Allen DZ, Challapalli S, McKee S et al. Impact of COVID-19 on nationwide pediatric otolaryngology: otitis media and myringotomy tube trends. *Am J Otolaryngol.* Mar-Apr 2022;43(2):103369. doi: 10.1016/j.amjoto.2021.103369.

COVID-19 information and guidance. Available at: https://www.yoifos.com/covid-19-information-and-guidance (accessed 31 January 2022).

ENT UK. Guidance for ENT during the COVID-19 pandemic. Available at: https://www.entuk.org/guidance-ent-during-covid-19-pandemic (accessed 31 January 2022).

Hobbs CV, Khaitan A, Kirmse BM, Borkowsky W. COVID-19 in children: a review and parallels to other hyperinflammatory syndromes. *Front Pediatr.* 2020;8:593455. doi: 10.3389/fped.2020.593455.

KEY POINTS

- COVID-19 is prevalent in children.
- It is associated with much lower morbidity than in adults.
- COVID-related fatalities in children are extremely rare.
- A very small number of children may present with a multisystem inflammatory picture.
- ORL organisations have been to the fore in producing effective guidelines for safe practice.
- The worldwide pandemic has brought about changes in ORL clinical practice, some of which look likely to persist.

INDEX

vascular compression 107
vascular masses 124
    nasal 81
    see also haemangiomas
vascular ring 107
VATER (VACTERL) association
    13, 106
velopharyngeal insufficiency 69
venous sinus thrombosis 22
ventilating facemask 3

vestibular clinics 60
vestibular neuronitis 60
viral infections
    acute otitis media 45
    causing facial palsy 64
    pharynx 67–8
    rhinosinusitis 84
visual reinforcement audiometry
    (VRA) 37
vocal cord nodules 113

vocal cord palsy 104, 113
voice disorders 113

Waardenburg's syndrome
    13, 32
waiting rooms 2
Waldeyer's ring 67
wheezing 99

X-linked disorders 32

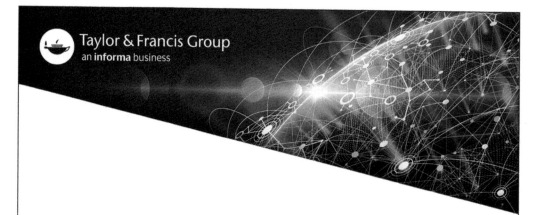
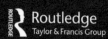
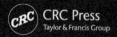

9781138579347